"Cancer is an increasingly common disease and one for which Chinese medicine is an important treatment option. Given that fact, it is a wonder there are so few well written books on the topic of integrative oncology. In this text, Drs. Giulio and Munson have offered Chinese medicine professionals a detailed examination of the topic, including the full range of Chinese medical therapies and how they can be applied clinically. Chapters contain information on rarely discussed treatments such as bloodletting, and are illustrated with short case narratives. All together this book should be an essential reference for anyone treating cancer patients."

Henry McCann, DAOM, L.Ac.

"This book is a long-anticipated contribution to the annals of traditional Chinese medicine-Western oncological concepts. A must have for any and all healthcare practitioners with an interest in integrative oncology who treat patients who have had, currently have, or are at risk of cancer. And frankly, we are all one degree separated from cancer."

Dennis von Elgg, L.Ac.

"I was so fortunate to be referred to doctors Munson and Di Giulio, who together pulled me back from the brink of total systemic collapse resulting from both lupus and stage-three breast cancer. I had massive immune and surgical complications from the aggressive Western medical treatment (chemotherapy, radiation, double mastectomy). They completely supported my system and alleviated my severe side effects with their incredible knowledge and application of Chinese medicine. Throughout my ordeal, I knew that as long as I could just climb up on their table, that I would enter another world for an hour where true healing was happening — both physical and spiritual. I absolutely credit their unfathomable talent, understanding and execution of Chinese medicine with my survival."

J.H.

"In the midst of my conventional medical treatments for breast cancer, it was a relief to be able to rest, recover, and get an integrative perspective on my prognosis and healing. Doctors Di Giulio and Munson eased my anxiety through their knowledge of cancer, conventional treatments, Eastern medicine, and nutrition. Their treatments reduced the side effects from surgery, chemotherapy and radiation and helped boost my immune system so that I could continue allopathic care without interruption. In the phase that followed, I recovered more quickly than expected. The remaining digestive issues, insomnia, menopausal symptoms, memory and concentration problems that I experienced as a result of my medical treatments resolved. It's hard to express just how emotionally and physically valuable it's been to have their compassionate and integrative care throughout this experience."

S.G.

Bridging the Gap

Integrative Oncology and the Practice of Traditional Chinese Medicine

Bianca Di Giulio, DAOM, L.Ac.
The Wellness Principle, USA

James Munson, DAOM, L.Ac.
Acupuncture and Oriental Medicine of Napa, USA

World Scientific

NEW JERSEY · LONDON · SINGAPORE · BEIJING · SHANGHAI · HONG KONG · TAIPEI · CHENNAI · TOKYO

Published by

World Scientific Publishing Co. Pte. Ltd.

5 Toh Tuck Link, Singapore 596224

USA office: 27 Warren Street, Suite 401-402, Hackensack, NJ 07601

UK office: 57 Shelton Street, Covent Garden, London WC2H 9HE

Library of Congress Cataloging-in-Publication Data

Names: Di Giulio, Bianca, author. | Munson, James (Acupuncturist), author.
Title: Bridging the gap : integrative oncology and the practice of
  traditional Chinese medicine / Bianca Di Giulio, James Munson.
Description: Hackensack, New Jersey : World Scientific, [2021] |
  Includes bibliographical references and index.
Identifiers: LCCN 2019053556 | ISBN 9789811204029 (hardcover) |
  ISBN 9789811204036 (ebook) | ISBN 9789811204036 (ebook other)
Subjects: MESH: Neoplasms--therapy | Integrative Oncology--methods |
  Medicine, Chinese Traditional--methods
Classification: LCC RC263 | NLM QZ 266 | DDC 616.99/4--dc23
LC record available at https://lccn.loc.gov/2019053556

British Library Cataloguing-in-Publication Data
A catalogue record for this book is available from the British Library.

With many thanks and gratitude to our editors and readers:
Emily Williams, Jessica Wakeman, Emily Hooker and Genevieve Di Giulio.

For any available supplementary material, please visit
https://www.worldscientific.com/worldscibooks/10.1142/11376#t=suppl

The authors dedicate this book to Mama Spice
and our muse,
Rufus aka Pork Chop.

Acknowledgments

"One looks back with appreciation to the brilliant teachers, but with gratitude to those who touched our human feelings. The curriculum is so much necessary raw material, but warmth is the vital element for the growing plant and for the soul of the child." — Carl Jung

I am forever grateful to my parents, Vito and Barbara Di Giulio, both brilliant educators who inspired curiosity and learning, while always encouraging me to follow my path.

Special thanks to my big sister, Genevieve, who has always provided endless support and love from day one of Chinese medicine school to this publication. She's the only one who let me needle her quite early on and is always willing to take my herbal formulas, as long as I don't tell her what's in them.

There are numerous teachers who have inspired my deep commitment and passion for Chinese medicine, but very special thanks to the following.

Amy Lee: Your generosity and sharing of information has no limits and I simply would not be where I am today without your guidance and mentorship, particularly in the field of integrative cancer care. Thank you for inspiring my curiosity about Chinese medicine oncology, enduring my endless questions over the years and always providing an answer.

Dennis von Elgg: Thank you for inspiring in me a true passion for Chinese herbal medicine. Your enthusiasm and brilliant teaching has guided me over the years, instilling a deep commitment to Chinese medicine that traverses beyond clinical frameworks.

Isaac Cohen: It is with heartfelt appreciation I thank you for your invaluable contributions to the field of Chinese medicine and integrative oncology. It has inspired so much of my research and clinical work. Thank you for being my doctoral advisor so many years ago and planting the seed that this book could become a reality.

Emily Hooker: From the first day of Chinese medicine school, through the thousands of hours of studying, exams and learning how to use a goniometer, your support has always been unwavering as a colleague and friend.

Dr. Di Giulio

I would not have been able to write, teach or provide treatment without the teaching or influence of so many. A few key people I would like to thank who influenced this book are:

My father, Tom Munson, my mother, Mary Ann Munson, my sisters, Cate and Mary, and brothers-in-law, Jeff Gutowski and Chris Ott for your continued love and support.

Ken Rose: Thank you for instilling the importance of approaching traditional Chinese medicine as a scholar-physician.

Robert Johns: Thank you for your steely commitment to the classics and instilling the importance of needling technique in me.

Pam Olson: Thank you for exemplifying the heart of a physician and your willingness to teach others.

Mark Frost: Thank you for your decades of commitment in teaching, providing treatment, and helping to rediscover the eight extraordinary meridians.

Yumiko Bamba: Thank you for elucidating the merit, importance and broad application of palpation and direct moxibustion.

Daniel Jiao: Thank you for providing me with an excellent foundation in traditional Chinese medicine herbalism.

Dr. James Munson

Contents

Prologue

"Maintaining order rather than correcting disorder is the ultimate principle of wisdom. To cure disease after it has appeared is like digging a well when one already feels thirsty or forging weapons after the war has already begun."

Neijing

"I ate a piece of cake a few weeks ago, and I'm sure that's why my cancer came back." Samantha sat across from me confessing this indulgence with wide eyes and an expression of fear and frustration. Just two years prior, Samantha was an energetic, vibrant young woman, successfully balancing a career and motherhood. Although recently divorced, a natural sense of optimism guided her toward a better life with her eight-year-old daughter. It was during this period of time that she began to experience unusual abdominal cramping and diarrhea after meals. At first thought, she attributed it to food poisoning, maybe a low-grade flu. The symptoms persisted beyond a few days and Samantha, being one never to ignore her health, went to her doctor. Having been given a diagnosis of gastritis, Samantha understood it would likely resolve within six weeks and left with an anti-diarrheal prescription. True to character, she followed the doctor's orders and trusted the symptoms would resolve. She was too busy in a new job and multitasking as a single mom to give these symptoms much attention otherwise. However, Samantha spent another few weeks in increasing discomfort; she found no relief from the abdominal pain and frequent loose stools. She later explained in my office, "Why would I have thought anything as absurd as cancer was the reason for my digestive problems?"

While Samantha's cancer journey was at its starting point, so was my Chinese medicine practice. Having completed the rigorous four-year didactic and clinical coursework, as well as passing national and state acupuncture board exams, I was an eager new apprentice to a seasoned Chinese medicine practitioner whose specialty was Chinese medical oncology. This was the gateway to a practice specialty I had never before considered. My exposure to cancer, both professionally and personally, was limited. Graduate schools emphasize the general practice of classical Chinese medicine, with almost half its coursework in Western medicine. After all, we are Eastern physicians practicing in a modern, Western-dominated medical paradigm. I was prepared for general practice. I was not prepared for oncology.

While I began post-graduate training, Samantha's symptoms worsened. Her appetite decreased and energy declined, but most notably her abdomen was hugely distended. She would recall, "It reminded me of being pregnant, but I knew I wasn't!" Several weeks later while still searching for answers, she returned to the doctor, who suggested irritable bowel syndrome, attributing this new diagnosis to stress related to navigating a new job and being a single-mother. This seemed logical enough. Samantha made attempts to manage her stress, watch her diet, and practice mindful meditation. Samantha had never experienced such an ongoing illness and was stubbornly intent on establishing the balance she assumed was lacking in her life in order to fully recover. However, the symptoms were relentless and eluded her. Despite conscious decision-making, time-management and a careful diet, her body further declined, and she felt increasing fatigue along with excruciating abdominal pain.

Not only did the discomfort and bloating persist, but it worsened to immeasurable levels. She later mentioned, "I went from seeming five-months pregnant to nine-months, in just a few weeks. I knew something was wrong." The third visit to the doctor's office led her to a gastroenterologist who recommended an endoscopy six-weeks later. She refused, not only because her capacity to endure the pain for several weeks longer was impossible, but intuitively, she knew it would not yield a correct diagnosis.

It was at this point, two months after the initial symptoms that Samantha asked if perhaps it was a gynecological concern. This question changed her life almost immediately. Within an hour, she met with her gynecologist. As Samantha recalls, "As soon as my gynecologist looked at my chart, and me, she knew what it was and sent me directly to the lab for ultrasound and blood work." Within twenty minutes of this appointment, six weeks after her initial digestive symptoms occurred, Samantha was diagnosed with stage IIIC ovarian cancer.

Samantha and I initially met after her diagnosis, staging and her conventional treatment plan was established. She was pleased her oncologist recommended acupuncture to address the side-effects of chemotherapy, which was scheduled to begin in two days. Samantha nervously sat across from me with palpable anxiety and uncertainty. She had not been to a Chinese medicine practitioner and understandably, she was not sure what to expect. As with most oncology patients, the "cancer-folder" was in one hand, no doubt full of medical records and treatment schedules, a pen in the other, thoroughly prepared to ask questions and take notes. Samantha was organized. This was in part personality, but also strengthened by her career as a social worker, trained to manage and navigate resources. She was determined to do everything possible to beat her diagnosis, and if that meant trying acupuncture, she would. I would learn not to expect anything less of her over the four years that she bravely journeyed through her cancer experience.

Samantha's story is not unique to modern day oncology. A patient seeks medical care and often presents with a myriad of physical symptoms that can create a bit of a guessing game for allopathic physicians. Stomach pain may be acid reflux, not a sign of gastrointestinal tumors; easy bruising and fatigue may only be anemia, not acute leukemia. Western physicians are questioned *ad nauseam* by patients wanting an immediate, accurate diagnosis from the minor to the complicated. One does not begin with an oncologist when there is abdominal bloating, nor should they. The phases of diagnosis have been predetermined by a framework and structure of care that physicians mandate and patients follow: first primary care, then specialty care. This was true of Samantha, digestive problems led her to her general physician, who referred her to gastroenterology, which led her to gynecology (by her own doing) and finally to oncology. It is from this point in her journey that Samantha's experience broadens from the singular, reductionist method of Western oncology, and into the expanse of integrative oncology, including multiple holistic therapies, like traditional Chinese medicine (TCM), which she powerfully harnessed to extend and improve her quality of life.

"So, you had a piece of cake for your daughter's birthday?" I remember responding to Samantha's panic-stricken statement. Her eyes were welling up, and she was visibly shaken. We both knew it was not merely one piece of cake that triggered the recurrence. She nodded, took a breath, but still began a discourse on how she knows sugar "feeds cancer" and negatively impacts the immune system. She expressed guilt for enjoying this one piece of cake, attributing it in part to her current circumstance. While we both recognized the link between sugar and cancer, it was apparent these concerns were merely superficial facts secondary to her fear and disappointment. Throughout the four years she was a patient, Samantha endured numerous cycles of chemotherapy, periods of remission and relapses. Through the depth of our established rapport between patient and provider, we knew, once again, we were about to embark on the next phase and progression of her disease. This would require more refinement and deeper integration of body, mind and spirit: the truest essence of Chinese medical oncology.

After listening patiently to her confession, I smiled and asked, "Was it at least chocolate cake?" Her eyes glistened with tears, but she grinned and said, "Well, of course." This early clinical experience with Samantha is imprinted in my mind, particularly as my career evolved from general practice with few oncology patients, to almost entirely TCM oncology. A vast majority of these patients had forged beyond the realm of Western medicine and were actively consulting with a myriad of complementary and alternative medicine providers to integrate with their conventional protocols. Samantha's cancer journey illustrates this dynamic as she developed her own integrative treatment plan that included Chinese herbal medicine, acupuncture, Naturopathy, Reiki, Energy Healing, oncology-specific nutrition and dietary programs alongside chemotherapy. Despite this amalgamation of healing therapies, there was no communication among the providers, and I was not an exception. Each healthcare professional diagnosed and treated according to their own scope, but this occurred separately and without a unified, collaborative plan. This seemed a significant disservice to our shared patient, contrary to the main principles of integrative medicine that emphasize a sharing of information based on therapeutic, patient-centered care.

Thus, as the number of individuals with cancer sought Chinese medicine, my curiosity to learn more about the disease itself from both a Western and Eastern perspective piqued. In order to dialogue with a range of medical professionals, it was necessary to become more informed and prepared to communicate effectively. The exploration led me directly to the practice of integrative oncology (IO), which afforded an opportunity to examine its structural foundation, concepts and with equal importance, the role of TCM within it. Here I discovered an immense discrepancy between the philosophical framework and ideology of IO with its practical application. Ultimately, this illustrated a need for true integration of TCM in modern oncology.

This is where the journey began.

Dr. Di Giulio

Foreword

We generally live in oblivion to what is actually happening to us. We rarely remember that we breathe, and we must do so, or have a heart-beat, which is obligatory for our life. We are happy with that silence. We notice it only when the silence is broken, by exertion or unfortunately through illness. Mostly, only then do we turn our attention to how the silence was broken. Medicine is the study that attempts to view and understand the silence, how it is broken and what can we do about restoring the silence or fixing what is broken.

Cancer is probably the best example of a disease that manifests many years following the initiation of the cancerous process, carcinogenesis, a process we still mostly don't understand. Nowadays, we diagnose many cancers because we screen for them through their silence with visual (mammograms or colonoscopies), molecular technologies (PSA for prostate cancer, or CA125 for ovarian cancer), or genetic analysis (BRCA gene mutation). When patients come to us with symptoms, and when finally we may diagnose the patient with cancer, for the most part these symptoms are not exclusive or specific to cancer, and frustrate patients, families and medical personnel alike. Cancer remains silent even when it rears its head.

The cancerous process from initiation, development and potential progression and spread (metastasis) involves invisible processes and interactions. Cancer is defined by cellular transformation (mutations), changes in shape (morphology), uncontrolled growth (neoplasia) and lack of obedience to structural and architectural determinism (invasion and metastasis). This description is fully modern, since we really didn't look at cells and defined their structural and molecular differences until recent decades. The technologies allowing us to interrogate cells, their parts and the substances that control their fate are all but modern. These processes take years to become visible even with the best of technical abilities.

As practitioners involved in cancer treatment and the care for patients with a cancer diagnosis, we learn another important lesson about medicine; the appreciation of time and the importance of vigilance. It takes many years to realize that immediate responses to treatment, like the complete elimination of a tumor, are only a suggestion to what might happen, and the fact that we cannot see or foresee what will happen next. With experience in cancer care comes a strange confidence in the need to attempt to translate the anxiety of the unknown and the anxiety of what we know might happen with practical vigilance. We generally view time as the progression from the past that happened, to the present that is, toward the future that will. In cancer vigilance we wish to transform the cause in the future, to change the past. This is a strange view of determinism. But, if we believe the only way to reverse the irreversible process of mutation in carcinogenesis is by elimination, we need to ask, elimination of what?

We now know how to harness and manipulate physiological processes such as the immune system and the endocrine system, or target cellular processes, such as growth and division signaling in the treatment of cancer. I remember just two decades ago when we were highly doubtful the immune system had anything to do with cancer control, while nowadays it is one of the only areas funded in cancer research. It is only three decades ago that we referred to cancer care as slash, burn and poison. Going back to my point above, we are still shy, arrogant and ignorant of what does it mean to eliminate cancer.

Chinese medicine developed a unique view of physiology, pathology and treatment modalities. Their system involved physiological concepts of invisible properties such as vitality, energy and spirit, viewed as both physical and non-physical. Or, organs that do not exist anatomically, such as the triple burner, or physiological functions ascribed to organs that do not correlate with our current view of organ functions, like ascribing metabolism to be mostly controlled by the spleen. Lack of instrumentation was not unique to Chinese medicine, and European medicine was modelled mostly after Greek tenets, although multiple empirical, non-theoretical practices co-existed. Plurality of practices with no theoretical coherence existed in China as well. When introduced to European anatomical and pathophysiological work from the 15th century on, Chinese scientists and physicians were divided as to how to reconcile the new knowledge with the traditional, or with the question whether they should all together abandon Chinese medicine.

In the early 20th century Chinese medicine was banned in China. Chinese medicine survived by a stroke of luck, when communist China faced the fulfilment of the promise to provide medicine to all, without a sufficient number of physicians or availability of medicines and facilities. Although the communists embraced the slogan of 'out with the old' and promised to follow only 'science and technology', they had no choice to at least temporarily keep and even promote Chinese medicine. In the Chinese experiment communism and nationalism merged, and Chinese medicine was now a source of national pride, and a subject for development. Scientific and clinical attempts to better describe the function, utility and modern basis of Chinese medicine were attempted with vigor. Again, an exuberant discussion developed between the traditionalists, who claimed Chinese medicine should be practiced as existed, with personalized tailoring of treatment and multiple component medicines, the modernizers, who wanted Chinese medicine to transform into modern medicine by examining the functionality and utility of the medical concepts and therapies under biomedical terms and the modernists who wanted to abandon Chinese medicine all together, attempting to show the superiority of biomedicine.

For three decades I tried to educate practitioners of Chinese medicine about the known, the imaginary, the wrong and mainly the unknown in cancer care, both Chinese and biomedical. I also tried to take the treasure 'buried in broad daylight' in the Chinese pharmacopeia to develop a new form of medicine based on traditional uses and functions and modern biomedical molecular functions. Merging my appreciation of science, with the belief, developed through clinical observation, that addressing multiple pathophysiological systems simultaneously is more akin to how the body works, and how we might get to the 'cause of the future' was an important attempt for the future of cancer care. I got frustrated with both. I never felt that I was a good teacher, and I was not able to secure funding for any of the new drugs, despite scientific success.

The current work is an attempt by two American practitioners of Chinese medicine, in the relatively narrow field of oncology, to describe their work and the utility found in the combined or exclusive use of Chinese medicine in cancer care. It is hard to shy away completely from the debates of superiority, or the attempts to find theoretical equivalence between tenets. Yet, it is clear that their experience and humanity in the approach to cancer care, including attempts to fulfill the multiple needs of our patients, beyond this or that specific indication, shines through. I remember the evolution of Chinese medicine in cancer care starting from a view that it is quackery, to not effective, to not scientific, to unknown potential side effects, to unknown interactions, to where it is today; no debate, just do what is accepted by the cancer establishment. I'm so happy to see that Dr. Di Giulio and Dr. Munson describe this current state in integrative oncology, and yet, take the clinical utility and application of the modalities employed in Chinese medicine to educate practitioners and patients of their usefulness. Hopefully this work will re-ignite a useful debate and provide the necessary funding, that is not just lip-service, or a method to anchor careers, to study various modalities with methodologies akin to them and the patience to follow the slowness of progress afforded to any biological science. More so, I hope this work will provide benefits to patients in need.

Isaac Cohen, DOM, Ph.D.
Oakland, CA
November 2019

Introduction

"It does not matter how slowly you go as long as you do not stop."

Confucius

The first question we are asked by cancer patients is, "What *can* Chinese medicine do for cancer?" As traditional Chinese medicine (TCM) doctors treating patients in various stages of this disease, we are familiar with this query but learning how to respond came carefully with time. Those who seek complementary therapy, like Chinese medicine, during their cancer experience, whether it is early diagnosis or in the midst of cyclical chemotherapy, are well-informed as to how conventional medicine will treat their cancer. What they are less familiar with is the breadth and scope of TCM oncology. Therefore, the question above is a pivotal moment for trained Oriental medicine practitioners to introduce this system of medicine that optimizes the body's ability to heal. Current statistics indicate that 1:2 men and 1:3 women will be diagnosed with cancer and over half will receive some form of complementary therapy.[1] This book aims to introduce the patient, caregiver, medical doctor or complementary healthcare provider to the valuable, rich therapy of TCM oncology. In addition, we hope to better prepare the Chinese medicine practitioner for the complexity of cancer management because it is likely that at some point every Chinese medicine practitioner will be sitting across from a cancer patient.

---

[1] Seely, 2012

This clinical preparation is an integral component to the Chinese medical profession and particularly crucial as the practice of IO gains momentum. It's philosophy is rooted in patient-centered care, with goals to reduce side effects of conventional treatment, improve quality of life and support emotional wellbeing. These outcomes are achieved through complementary therapies including acupuncture, bodywork, naturopathic medicine, and meditation to name a few. While patient empowerment is central to this subject, the spectrum of care is structured around evidence-based medicine as an adjunct to Western oncology protocols. As such, modalities such as moxibustion that do not meet the rigid scientific standards set forth by the medical community are often discouraged or dismissed as not having therapeutic value. Acupuncture, however, has been researched endlessly and with enough scrutiny that it is an accepted form of supportive therapy.

An extremely thorough systematic review of integrative oncology programs worldwide found that an increasing number of multifaceted facilities exist. Out of the 29 sites reviewed, acupuncture is offered at 41% of these locations.[2] There is reference to "Traditional Chinese Medicine" as an offered service, but it falls in less than 2% of program centers.[3] We can conclude that moxibustion, Chinese dietary therapy and herbal medicine are subsequently not available, indicating the limited degree to which the full-spectrum of what TCM offers is presented. Despite the breadth and longevity of the medicine, harnessed by a vast range of therapeutic abilities, the reality is that TCM practitioners limit their scope when it comes to integrative cancer care. The cause for this trend can be linked to several identifiable factors.

The barriers to seamless collaboration among holistic and conventional medical doctors are extensive. In cancer management, these challenges are acutely present and frequently frustrating. Communication among oncologists and natural medicine doctors is influenced by several factors. For example, it becomes difficult to dialogue as a collaborative unit when there is not a shared facility. The same systematic review noted above found that only 41% of the IO centers offer conventional treatments

---

[2] Seely, 2012
[3] ibid

and complementary therapies in the same location. In private practice, patients are either self-referred based on a personal recommendation or another healthcare provider suggested acupuncture to alleviate side effects. It is rare to receive a note, email, or call from an oncologist to discuss patient care. A survey of Chinese medicine practices in Northern California demonstrated these findings by reporting that only 2% of TCM providers were consulted by a biomedical physician.[4] In contrast, of the same respondents only 8% reported they *always* initiate communication. Thus, illustrating a lack of dialogue among all providers involved in the patient's care and an opportunity to improve this collaborative dynamic.

The disconnect between doctors, as well as with patients, diminishes the therapeutic value of Chinese medicine before it can even begin, causing practitioners to limit their practice approaches and submit to basic, palliative protocols. This is not to say that focusing on improving the quality of life before, during or after cancer treatment is without importance or purpose. However, this resignation to solely mitigate side-effects of allopathic treatment compromises the integrity of the profession and stunts the advancement of Chinese medicine in a modern medical world. This became the turning point in our clinical focus, choosing to explore beyond the safe nest of private practice to search for collaborative relationships among cancer management providers. We cautiously hoped to discover integrative philosophies that respectfully valued our medicine and vice-versa.

We quickly discovered that although a common vision of whole-person, patient-centered medicine is shared among integrative oncology systems, the methods and applications are diverse. The role and placement of Chinese medicine therapies was largely limited to acupuncture. We began to question how the concept of integrative oncology was truly integrative, which lead to the purpose of this book. First, we wish to present the current definitions and terrains of integrative oncology, as well as identify how Chinese medicine is practiced within them. This introduces the reader into the dynamics of integrated medicine and the obstacles Eastern doctors face despite attempts to collaborate care for the health of a shared patient. Second, as traditional medicine practitioners who have learned from the long line of teachers that come before us, we inherently value the sharing

---

[4] Abrams et al., 2009

of concepts, clinical applications and humbly contribute to the evolution of Chinese medicine for new students or seasoned practitioners seeking to learn and apply these approaches.

The most significant obstacle TCM practitioners contend with, which is introduced early in Chinese medical education, is a legal consideration. By law, a provider who is not a licensed oncologist cannot treat cancer. The risk of a malpractice lawsuit leads very few TCM practitioners to claim that treatment goals are to "treat cancer." The survey of licensed acupuncturists again sheds light on this issue with just 32% reporting they utilize TCM to treat the cancer itself.[5] The study did not indicate why providers choose not to treat the cancer, and while a myriad of possibilities can be imagined, we reason the main impediment is related to legality. So, although Chinese medical schools educate students on the properties of certain herbs, like *bai hua she she cao* (oldenlandia diffusa), that have antineoplastic effects in high concentrations, it is prohibited for that purpose. Similarly, many patients have been told by their oncologists not to continue acupuncture if there is risk of infection due to neutropenia, a condition of low white blood cells. More frequently than not, patients heed this warning from their doctor and TCM treatments are postponed. Ironically, this is precisely the time when Chinese medicine can increase white blood cells and immunity by careful and regular application of moxibustion, as well as herbal medicine and nutritional recommendations. This is another window of opportunity for our profession to educate and inform the patient and, if possible, the doctor, to not compromise the safe, therapeutic capacity of this medicine.

As our journey into this specialty evolved we became acutely aware it is not only Western medical facilities that have singled out acupuncture (above other TCM modalities) exclusively for the purpose of cancer management. It appears also, classically-trained acupuncturists in private practice tend to rely solely on needling treatments for cancer patients. There may be minimal inclusion of indirect moxibustion on ST-36 (*zu san li*) for immunity, but rarely have we observed more than this. This is not to say these techniques are irrelevant, as acupuncture is inherently valuable in its ability to lessen symptoms of nausea, vomiting, fatigue or pain as a

---

[5] Abrams et al., 2009

result of conventional oncology treatments. For the purpose of this topic, we again refer to the survey of over 400 TCM practitioners who reported that of the modalities that encompass Chinese medicine, including moxibustion, herbal prescription, dietary advice and exercise, acupuncture was used by 98% of the practitioners and regarded as the most useful for oncology patients.[6] By comparison, moxibustion was used by 17.3% for cancer care and dietary advice was a mere 35%.[7] This imbalance must be remedied. As doctors of Chinese medicine, the onus of understanding and incorporating multiple modalities to treat disease is upon us. The individual components of TCM are like spokes on a wheel, which give it strength and balance. Without all the spokes, there is still a functional wheel that serves a purpose, but the structural integrity of the wheel is compromised. With all of the spokes to balance the wheel, it is stronger, more efficient, and leads to a faster desired destination.

The importance of being a well-rounded practitioner with respect to being adept at all the major modalities in TCM is consistently repeated throughout Chinese medical literature. Classical scholar of such texts, Paul U. Unschuld identifies this concept in at least four chapters of the *Su Wen*, the seminal text of Chinese medicine. He delves into this idea confirming the integral value of multifaceted skills and techniques. From the message of *Su Wen* Chapter 12, he reflects, "To be unaware of even one of these approaches is to be unable to confront the advance of a disease at all stages of its development..."[8] The wheel must be complete, the spokes equally important to the mechanism in order to optimize its function and outcome. A superb excerpt from *Su Wen* Chapter 24 clearly illustrates how physicians were committed to the breadth of therapeutic modalities[9]:

> "When the physical appearance is joyful, while the mind suffers, the disease emerges in the vessels. Treat it with cauterization and piercing. When the physical appearance is joyful and the mind is joyful [too], the disease emerges in the flesh. Treat it with needles and [pointed] stones. When the physical

---

[6] Abrams et al., 2009

[7] ibid

[8] Unschuld, 2003

[9] ibid

appearance suffers while the mind is joyful, the disease emerges in the sinews. Treat it with poultice and stretching [exercises]. When the physical appearance suffers and the mind suffers [too], the disease emerges in the gullet and in the throat. Treat it with the one hundred drugs."

In this passage we can identify multiple approaches employed by the doctor according to disease presentation, interestingly in both body and mind. Cauterization refers to burning, which we correlate now to modern day direct moxibustion or heat therapy. Piercing is referenced and akin to modern day needling technique known as pricking therapy or bloodletting. The needles used in this early form of acupuncture were made of sharp stones. Poultices maintain a long history in any era or region of medicine, used as topical herbal remedies. In this passage, exercise is referred to as stretching, an invaluable modality practitioners must also encourage in moderate amounts for cancer patients. As dedicated doctors of this system of medicine, we feel called to contribute and offer clinical guidelines for true integrative medicine practices that macro-level institutions may employ, as well as the clinician in private practice. We must become masters of the modalities, as the medicine intends.

It is for this reason an overview of the history of Chinese medicine oncology is where our book begins, inviting the reader to dig a bit deeper, delve into the classical texts that are our timeless teachers. Whether for the uninitiated person who wishes to learn more about medicine of the East, the TCM student, or seasoned practitioner, returning to the root of the medicine is valid and necessary. While this can be a laborious task as a reader, particularly for the clinician wanting to skip over the scientific history and behavior of a disease and get straight into treatment approaches, we encourage the reader to familiarize oneself with the historical framework of cancer. TCM is a practice that has evolved and refined itself over thousands of years. Its inception began with the *Huang Di Nei Jing*, composed during the Han Dynasty (206 B.C.E.-220 C.E.). It is a compilation of two texts, *Su Wen* and *Ling Shu*, both integral to the foundation, principles and techniques we embrace today. Modern Chinese medicine doctors can treat a wide variety of diseases because of these classical works. The principles of *yin-yang* theory, excess and deficient, interior and exterior, cold or hot are as timeless as the texts they are presented in, profoundly capable of being applied to the common cold or cancer. While Chinese medicine is not considered "evidence-based," its foundation is unchanged nor has it wavered since its development, unlike the practice of modern, reductionist Western medicine. Chinese medical therapies are able to adapt to biomedical advancements. Its flexible nature allows itself to interpret modern medicine into its own constructs to yield successful therapeutic outcomes.

From the discourse of the East, we briefly shift our historical lens to the West. Just as physicians in the ancient East observed and treated various malignancies, so did the doctors in the West. The famous physician Hippocrates known as the "father of medicine," played an integral role in early cancer theory and diagnosis. His primary hypothesis on the cause of cancer was explained by the concept of the four humors or body fluids: blood, phlegm, yellow and black bile. He theorized that disease developed due to an imbalance of these substances. This interpretation of disease correlates to Chinese medicine's early understanding of tumor formation and pathogenic causes. Historical insights such as these will be explored and are particularly interesting when juxtaposing early cancer theories, treatments and diagnoses of both medical cultures.

The individual historical perspectives serve as a vantage point in our assessment of integrative oncology practices. This overview derives from experiences as doctoral interns in IO facilities, mentorships with licensed medical doctors, oncology dieticians and complimentary cancer providers. These professional opportunities were significant to the development of this material, enabling a bird's eye view of integrative medicine. We do not intend to outline numerous discrepancies of IO programs, as we are equally indebted to modern medicine capabilities. At this point in biomedicine, we must rely upon conventional therapies as they provide the possibility of curing aggressive diseases like cancer. Our scope of practice is greatly limited in the West, and while measures toward integration are happening, they are dictated by science and sadly, Chinese medicine is not recognized as such at this time. Fortunately, however, we hold the tools to mitigate the harsh cytotoxic effects of chemotherapeutic agents, radiation, pharmaceutical side-effects, as well as addressing the emotional terrain of cancer diagnosis. Chinese medicine practitioners who commit to this endeavor, with skill, focus and determination can facilitate innate healing of the individual, optimizing the body's capacity to fight the cancer and essentially, treat it.

For licensed practitioners, this serves as a jumping off point into clinical guidelines. We chose not to divide the content of this book by cancer type. Our goal is to highlight each modality that comprises Chinese medicine, building upon each pillar to create a foundation of clinical understanding and therapeutic purpose for refined cancer management. This enables the clinician to reference specific modalities as appropriate, and in that way become more comfortable integrating the medicine. We begin with the core elements of diagnosis in TCM oncology. From this vantage point a pathway into acupuncture therapy, Chinese herbal medicine, diet, exercise and manual therapy is illuminated. As with everything in Chinese medicine we also must reflect on the *shen*, or spirit. Its relationship to disease is deeply rooted in the constitution and, we feel, cannot be ignored in cancer care. Consequently, we are committed to the system of the eight-extraordinary meridians (EEM) to address emotional complexities of the cancer experience. As the famous Chinese physician, Li Shi-Zhen once stated, "If physicians are not aware of such theories of the extraordinary channels, they will remain in the dark as to the cause of disease."[10]

Additionally, as students of Chinese medicine and novice practitioners who knew very little about oncology, we struggled extensively in learning how best to begin an intake with a cancer patient. There were no guidelines that integrated our knowledge of Chinese medicine with Western oncology. We aim to rectify that situation by presenting a framework for a basic TCM oncology intake that the licensed practitioner can modify. This enables seamless coordination with the patient's conventional cancer treatment plan in order to treat the physical and emotional side-effects, concurrent health issues and encourage collaboration among providers. All of these components to integrative cancer care will be presented in case studies from our clinical experience to demonstrate the capacity of Chinese medicine, the value of using it as a system with multiple modalities at play and emphasizing its merit in integrative oncology. It is in this spirit of sharing, challenging concepts and methods while contributing to the evolution of health and wellness that we write this book.

---

[10] Chase et al., 2010

References

Abrams, D. I., & Weil, A. (2009). *Integrative Oncology*. New York, NY: Oxford University Press.

Chace, C., & Shima, M. (2010). *An Exposition on the Eight Extraordinary Vessels*. Seattle, Washington: Eastland press.

Seely, D., & Young, S. (2012). *A Systematic Review of Integrative Oncology Programs*. Retrieved September 10, 2018, from http://www.current-oncology.com/index.php/oncology/article/view/1182/1078

Unschuld, P. U. (2003). *Huang Di Nei Jing Su Wen: Nature, knowledge, imagery in an ancient Chinese medical text: With an appendix, the doctrine of the five periods and six qi in the Huang Di Nei Jing Su Wen*. Berkeley, CA: University of California Press.

1 What is Integrative Oncology?

"A doctor, like anyone else who has to deal with human beings, each of them unique, cannot be a scientist; he is either, like the surgeon, a craftsman, or, like the physician and the psychologist, an artist."

W.H. Auden

Cancer is a complex condition encompassing hundreds of diseases within its presentation. Its characteristics are extensive, ranging from slow cellular division to fast, aggressive proliferation. The potency of this ever-evolving disease necessitates innovative and integrative therapies. The philosophy of IO was born from this awareness, a commitment to science and evidence-based medicine, while also recognizing therapeutic value in complementary modalities like traditional Chinese medicine. IO advocates conceptualize a framework of collaboration among medical paradigms to achieve a curable outcome that empowers the patient as well as the body's ability to heal. The symbiotic energy of both the cause (cancer) and the effect (IO) harness the focus of Western and complementary medical systems due to its complex nature. This investigation is ideally done alongside patients and their loved ones to explore the capacity of healing through integrative approaches. As a result, IO practices are further empowered by the disease it seeks to manage and because of this, therapies outside the scope of conventional medicine are becoming implemented in the clinical environment.

For practitioners of Chinese medicine this is good news. At the forefront of the evolution of integrative medicine in the West, we are participants in early waves of collaborative treatment approaches that implement a range of complementary modalities alongside biomedicine. This is occurring at small public health clinics and also at large private hospitals where a range of services are valued and accepted more than ever before. Consequently, there is a momentous opportunity to bridge the gap between medicine of the West and the East. But building this bridge does not come seamlessly and without its challenges. Add in the complexity of a disease like cancer and the guidelines of integration become even more convoluted. As doctors of TCM, we honed our skills in Chinese medical oncology. It appeared only natural to lean into IO and explore its parameters, curious about the role of Chinese medicine within it.

We posed two simple questions as we embarked on this exploration. First, where does IO originate? In Chinese medicine diagnosis, the root must be examined to understand the branch. Its history would impart perspective on its evolutionary process as a prominent figure in the multitude of cancer management techniques. Secondly, what is the agreed upon definition of IO? Ideally, this clearly elucidates IO's core mission and with equal importance, to inform complementary providers, like us, the degree to which Chinese medicine may or may not be an equal part to a greater whole. The simplicity of these queries unveiled the incredible complexity of this specialty. In a relatively brief period of time, as a result of on-site internships and doctoral research that analyzed IO programs, it became clear that the ideology of collaborative cancer care is inherently different from clinical applications at the ground level.

The Origins: Integrative Medicine

Every modality of medicine can be traced back to its historical origins, a link to the natural evolutionary processes that occur through experience, time, and sharing of information that led to its maturation. Integrative medicine is an example of this. It is an illustration of scientific advancement combined with perspectives that acknowledge the whole body, relating physical and emotional elements with disease presentation. This movement has gained significant momentum within the last few decades in the West as individuals grow increasingly frustrated with healthcare systems that appear depersonalized by doctors who have limited interaction time with patients and seem to follow medical flow-charts to reach diagnoses and treatment strategies. In our clinical experience, this is often what we hear from new patients who express their frustration stating, "My doctor can't do anything except prescribe anti-inflammatories for the pain, so I thought I'd try acupuncture."

Time and again we consult with individuals seeking complementary modalities to achieve health goals through more natural means and quite simply, conventional medicine struggles to meet these demands. We highly regard this patient curiosity because it empowers individuals to actively participate in their own health and wellness, from illness prevention to recovery. Thus, the limits of allopathic medicine to treat the whole person, dissatisfaction with standard medical care, and a burgeoning field of mind-body medicine shifted the healthcare paradigm. Patients created their own integrative health system by blending a myriad of disciplines: physical exams with their primary physician, access to medication and emergency services, in combination with holistic, natural medicine to address chronic, underlying conditions that encompass the whole person. Naturally, this resulted in integrative medicine (IM) designs that generated a following by larger health institutions, which incorporated mind-body modalities, like yoga or meditation. These early inroads of medical integration provided a refreshing perspective on medicine, an improved outlook on wellness and empowered individuals to do more than merely "take their medicine and call the doctor."

It is not surprising that subspecialties were born from the foundation of IM. It is even less astonishing that integrative approaches surfaced in the field of oncology. While there are no exact origins of integrative medicine, nor can we link its popularity to a particular individual or institution, there are certainly major influencers, such as Dr. Andrew Weil. Dr. Weil is a classically trained Western medical doctor who pioneered early efforts to align allopathic and holistic medicine. One of the earliest publications on the topic of integrated cancer treatment is co-authored with IO proponent Dr. Donald Abrams. In their book entitled, *Integrative Oncology*, Dr. Weil outlines the fundamental components that embody an ideal relationship between medical paradigms. He states, "Integrative medicine does include ideas and practices currently beyond the scope of the conventional, but it neither accepts conventional therapies nor accept alternative ones uncritically. And it emphasizes principles that may or may not be associated with CAM (complementary and alternative medicine)."[11] Four major tenets are proposed as part of the integrative medical model proposed by Dr. Weil:

- The natural healing power of the organism
- Whole person medicine
- The importance of lifestyle
- The critical role of the doctor-patient relationship[12]

This viewpoint delineates central characteristics of IM and essentially sets the stage for Western trained physicians to approach patient healthcare and the treatment of disease with strategies that extend beyond linear medicine. These core values illuminate the future landscape of integrated healthcare. It recognizes the individual as a whole system, beyond quantitative measurements based in reductionist biomedical theory to diagnose and treat illness.

The IM principles noted above are embedded in the rich clinical history of Chinese medicine, which was developed thousands of years ago. These core values are not new to those trained in Chinese medicine. They are as inherent to the practice as *yin-yang* theory. The TCM physician observes disease as a result of imbalance through any combination of vital substances, energy and physiology. The ability to discern the cause of illness results from diagnostic skills that take into account the entire constitution, the whole person. There is no separation within the living organism, and through specialized skill and techniques, TCM optimizes the organism to heal itself. In order to support the body to restore health, the physician utilizes multiple pillars and techniques of the medicine to advise the patient on diet, lifestyle and emotional wellness. Thus, integrative medicine was happening long before modern definitions of it. And yet, because our medical philosophy aligns with Eastern traditions in a Western dominated medical system, Chinese medicine remains heavily scrutinized as researchers

---

[11] Weil, Abrams
[12] ibid

seek definitive scientific explanations for how it works, instead of trusting its empirical research and dynamic medical scope.

This reluctance provides insight into Chinese medicine's limited position in the IO specialty. Is it science or merely an esoteric medical art? It is a great question, some say debate, in our profession as to whether TCM is art or science. If it is the former, the likelihood the entire system of Chinese medicine is ever entirely welcomed into open, allopathic arms is slim. Within the spectrum of Western standards, TCM is not a science, given a deficiency of evidence-based results that indicate clear measurements of success. In a seminal book about Chinese medicine, *The Web That Has No Weaver*, Dr. Ted Kaptchuk aptly addresses this idea stating, "If we mean by science the relatively recent intellectual and technological development in the West, Chinese medicine is not scientific. It is instead a prescientific tradition that has survived into the modern age and remains another way of doing things. But it does resemble science in that it is grounded in conscientious observation, of phenomena, guided by rational, logically consistent, and communicable thought process."[13] In this construct Chinese medicine, true to its nature, weaves among philosophies of medicine as art and among the confines of medicine rooted in science.

Whichever perception of TCM, science-based medicine leads the charge in the West. Double-blind, randomized studies determine standards of medical intervention, but Chinese medicine is a system that cannot be measured according to these rigid scientific criteria. While there are numerous studies that demonstrate its potential (namely acupuncture), it remains under the microscope, cautiously accepted and subject to Western clinical guidelines. The outcome has resulted in treatments that employ only technical methods of acupuncture therapy for acute patterns or with respect to oncology, palliative care. This is evident in integrative medical facilities that hire licensed acupuncturists and only permit needle-based treatments to address nausea, fatigue or cancer-related pain and prohibit the range of diagnostic methods or techniques integral to TCM. This grossly limits the capacity of Chinese medicine. These barriers will be further explored in this chapter, but first

---

[13] Kaptchuck, 2008

we follow the path from the foundation of IM philosophy into the vast realm of integrative oncology.

From Integrative Medicine, To Integrative Oncology

The endeavor to explore the culture of IO began in 2013 as a byproduct of doctoral research in Chinese medical oncology and a growing specialty in cancer. Even before pursuing a doctorate in TCM, there was a palpable energy emanating from our cancer patients who used the buzzword "integrative oncology" with hope and expectation. While much can be assumed from the terminology and inferred through professional experience, it still required closer analysis. Thus, having focused entirely on the history, evolution, principles and treatment of cancer from a TCM viewpoint, it was only natural to juxtapose this same data to conventional oncology. This examination reviewed the parameters of this multidisciplinary medical approach, carefully peeling the layers away from the ideology of collaborative medicine in order to glimpse at actual practices where the role of Chinese medicine was more closely scrutinized.

The process of discovering a unified definition of IO unveiled extensive interpretations that spanned from prominent cancer hospitals to private clinics. A proponent of collaborative medicine, Dr. Stephen Sagar explains the discipline as, "…both a science and a philosophy that focuses on the complexity of the health of cancer patients and proposes a multitude of approaches to accompany the conventional therapies of surgery, chemotherapy, molecular therapeutics, and radiotherapy to facilitate health."[14] In addition, Dr. Sagar points out that IO philosophy encompasses socio-cultural components to care, recognizing such implications that influence decision-making, as well as access to self-empowering resources that are financially stable, safe and that improve outcomes. This reflects a very real concern in the spectrum of oncology familiar to allopathic and complementary doctors alike: cancer patients are seeking curative outcomes and the diagnosis has the potential to lead vulnerable patients toward therapies that are possibly dangerous, ineffective and carry a hefty price tag.

---

[14] Sagar, 2008

For example, we consulted with a patient diagnosed with stage III colon cancer actively seeking a multitude of opinions following a surgical resection. His oncologist prescribed chemotherapy to treat the remaining cancer cells, but this patient refused, expressing a deep, visceral response to allowing "toxic medicine" into his body. Point blank, he asked if Chinese medicine could cure his cancer. This question provides the TCM doctor with an immense opportunity that benefits the patient in two ways. First, recognize that in this specific case the patient was seeking a fast, straightforward cure. Medical ethics override any discourse that insinuates Chinese medicine as a singular therapy to quickly eradicate his cancer cells. But this also opened a dialogue that informed him about the principles of Chinese medicine oncology for cancer management, and how it integrates with conventional treatments from acupuncture and moxibustion to herbal medicine. At the follow-up appointment, he shared his decision to opt for an alternative therapy at an "integrative cancer center" even though it was extremely costly and not covered by insurance. His understanding of the treatment was vague, but he was compelled by the case manager who reviewed his diagnosis and proposed the course of treatment. He was told "in two months you'll be cured." We asked questions about this protocol to determine its potential harm or efficacy and explore its parameters. However, he was uncertain as to what medicine, vitamins or supplements he would be treated with for those two months.

The outcome of this case is unknown, as the patient proceeded with the alternative therapy and did not follow-up. These interactions occur in TCM cancer management, and patients should feel empowered to ask questions, seek multiple opinions and ultimately make the best choice for themselves. Of equal regard, however, is the integrity of the clinician to listen and inform the patient within their scope of practice. The clinician's role should never be to exploit or promise a healing outcome. An integral strength of Chinese medicine is its duality to observe the whole person, diagnose according to constitution and deliver medicine through skilled treatment protocols, which optimize the healing process. And in some cases, this aligns with curable outcomes as a result of balanced integration. This is the message we share with cancer patients.

This patient's interaction provides insight as to why a singular, agreed upon definition of IO did not exist for many years. Countless medical disciplines and providers in cancer care had the autonomy to label a particular therapy or practice as "integrative" regardless of proven, therapeutic efficacy. Thus, the merge of a multitude of modalities interconnected to the framework of conventional medicine lead to variable interpretations of IO. What ensued was an ambiguous medical melting pot that ultimately impacts those navigating collaborative treatments. In response to this confusion, as well as an apparent demand by cancer patients seeking complementary therapies, the Society of Integrative Oncology (SIO) was established in 2003.

The SIO platform promotes communication among cancer providers, including classically-trained Western physicians, practitioners of Eastern medicine, naturopathic doctors, massage therapists, herbalists, social workers and professionals committed to cancer management and recovery. It is instrumental in the advancement of multidisciplinary systems of care. Regardless of discipline, members share a common goal that promotes evidence-based standards of integrative oncology. It proposes an awareness and sensitivity of the patient's mental, emotional and spiritual wellness, while combining mainstream care and complementary therapies to treat the whole person.

The management of cancer requires a delicate balance of interventions focusing on two simple principles of equal measure: eradication of the disease and optimizing the body's innate ability to heal. Biomedicine takes the role of "attack therapy" directed at the cancer cells, while complementary modalities aim to strengthen the cancer patient and potentiate healing. Illustrating these methods of integration are renowned cancer hospitals, such as Memorial Sloan Kettering Cancer Center (MSKCC), MD Anderson Cancer Center, Mayo Clinic, and Cancer Treatment Centers of America (CTCA). Each facility has implemented IO programs that encompass these elements of care reflected in its language, distinctive structure and tone, which are demonstrated by a wide variety of therapies and how they are defined. The most common modalities include acupuncture, mind-body medicine, yoga, *Qigong*, massage therapy, and nutritional and dietary advice. Despite the myriad differences among them, the philosophy of IO weaves through a system that is centralized around conventional medicine protocols, such as chemotherapy, radiation and surgery, which all may be supported by adjunctive therapies. With equal, if not greater value, is the premise that IO practices are founded in evidence-based medicine and scientific findings.

This philosophy is evident in a growing number of hospitals implementing IO practices. Program features display a variety of therapies and services that demonstrate the aspects of the integrative oncology paradigm. For example, the University of Texas MD Anderson Cancer Center offers therapeutic modalities such as acupuncture stating, "*The Integrative Medicine Program* engages patients and their families to become active participants in improving their physical, psycho-spiritual and social health. The ultimate goals are to optimize health, quality of life and clinical outcomes through personalized evidence-based clinical care, exceptional research and education. We provide access to multiple databases of authoritative, up-to-date reviews on the evidence and safety for the use of herbs, supplements, vitamins, and minerals, as well as other complementary medicine modalities."[15]

The MD Anderson IM program was established in 1998 and is one of the earliest models of collaborative cancer care. A brief overview of their program characteristics will demonstrate standard clinical integration common to IO centers. The gateway to adjunctive therapy options begins with a consultation led by a Western-trained doctor who outlines various modalities, reviewing the benefits and risks. Nutritional counseling, oncology massage, exercise therapy, meditation, health psychology, music therapy and acupuncture are examples of services cancer patients may access upon physician approval. The primary function of these supportive modalities is to reduce side-effects of conventional medicine, improve quality of life, mental outlook, and optimize outcomes. IM practitioners collaborate weekly to review cases, devise treatment plans and maintain shared access to patient records.[16] Its framework offers elements of integrative, patient-centered care in the management of cancer.

Closer examination of Chinese medicine's role within this structure indicates vast therapeutic limitations. First, acupuncture is the only modality of TCM offered at MD Anderson. The literature explains its function is to reduce side-effects related to conventional medicine, such as neuropathy, hot flashes or dry mouth, and it also can promote well-being to alleviate

---

[15] MD Anderson Cancer Center, 2018
[16] Seely, 2012

stress.[17] While acupuncture is effective for those ailments and should not be discounted, there is a significant lack of detail about the system of Chinese medicine. Yes, acupuncture addresses acute physical side-effects, but this occurs as the therapeutic outcome after diagnostic assessment of the whole person. The insertion of needles according to simple point indications grossly undermines the capacity of the medicine. A comprehensive diagnosis enables the practitioner to treat the symptoms, what is referred to as the branch in TCM, and simultaneously address the root, or underlying condition.

Unfortunately, this does not appear to be happening at the ground level. In October 2018, a news source for all things TCM, *Acupuncture Today* interviewed a licensed acupuncturist employed at the integrative medical center of MD Anderson. On the periphery, the picture of acupuncture as part of the integrative oncology model appears collaborative. Each practitioner treats 30–50 cancer patients per week, and clinical staff participates in interdisciplinary meetings to review cases. According to the source, "At these meetings, as an acupuncturist, I can openly discuss the pathology of cancer in Eastern medicine terms and share different ways we can intervene."[18] When acupuncture therapy is the only modality at the disposal of a trained Chinese medicine physician, what are the remaining interventions possible? The interview proudly highlights this union of disciplines, but in doing so, it also unveils definitive boundaries within its integration. These are evident in the following ways:

- Acupuncture therapy first requires pre-authorization by a medical doctor
- Development of the integrated treatment plan does not include the licensed acupuncturist's presence and professional input
- Herbal recommendations or formulas are not permitted
- Moxibustion therapy is not allowed

The guidelines and procedures set forth demonstrate how the Chinese medicine practitioner is merely a technician. Such facts, again, illustrate a

---

[17] MD Anderson, Acupuncture, 2018
[18] Reddy, 2018

real discrepancy in the integrative paradigm. The merge of disciplines is also made clear by the practitioner's approach to the language of medicine. The practitioner in the interview asserts that acupuncturists must consider their role in integrative hospitals as providers responsible for acclimating to the Western medical environment. It is upon us to bridge the gap, communicate on their terms and weave into conventional standards. As an example, he suggests, "…instead of discussing *Qi* with a medical team, we should speak more of how acupuncture can affect the production of endogenous opioids or reduce inflammation. Instead of relying solely on pulse and tongue, looking through MRI/CT or PET scan to gain intimate knowledge of tumor location or surgical changes is essential."[19]

Chinese medicine doctors should be familiar with Western biomedicine, cancer diagnosis, tumor pathology and treatments. The ability to dialogue with an oncologist is necessary, and providers must become well-versed in the medical vocabulary associated with neoplastic disease. In modern medicine, there is always an opportunity to translate our terminology in order to clarify its purpose. We argue, however, that if the ideology of integrative oncology relies upon collaboration and equal regard for other disciplines, then Western physicians must also learn our language as well. This goes beyond palliative care referrals. We are inviting our colleagues into the medical acumen of Chinese medicine.

The program at MD Anderson Cancer Center is one example of an integrative oncology model. From this established perspective, we present a brief comparative analysis of an equally renowned cancer hospital, Memorial Sloan Kettering Cancer Center (MSKCC). Between the two reputable facilities, there are obvious overlaps and similar philosophy toward integrative practices. MSKCC has designed a broad integrative department that promotes multidisciplinary avenues in cancer management. In addition to program offerings, it is a leading research institution. As such, it has carved a pathway enabling greater access to complementary therapies alongside conventional treatments. Cancer patients consult with a physician or nurse specialist to coordinate an "integrative care plan,"[20] and patient records are shared among disciplines. The IM model is well-designed with a multitude

---

[19] Reddy, 2018
[20] MSKCC, 2018

of classes, workshops and services available to cancer patients. Individual therapies include acupuncture, both private and community style, as well as Swedish, deep tissue, or lymphedema massage. Mind-body therapies, medical *Qigong*, Reiki and Shiatsu are also available. All of these are fee-for-service, on-site at the IM facility.

The indications promoting the use of acupuncture for cancer and its related symptoms align with those previously noted at MD Anderson. They emphasize palliative care protocols to reduce side-effects that correlate to the disease or conventional treatment. An equally short description of acupuncture, MSKCC notes it is a form of traditional Chinese medicine validated by science through its ability to "...stimulate the nervous system to release certain chemicals in the brain."[21] This highlights a challenge Chinese medicine contends with in modern medicine. It gains relevance when validated by scientific methods, ushered into programs only after having determined its efficacy as safe and nonthreatening. However, this message does not encompass an integrated viewpoint. It leans West and into scientific interpretations. This discounts thousands of years of empirical research and methodology engraved in TCM. So, the Chinese medicine profession is caught between both paradigms, science and art. While this may appear to be self-limiting and an undesirable position for the profession, it actually illustrates the flexible nature of Eastern medicine to evolve alongside our conventional colleagues, as well as the disease itself.

How does this flexibility occur? Quite simply, the field of TCM has the benefit of an extremely well-rounded education. Practitioners adhere to classical texts, relying upon empirical research of physicians more than three-thousand years ago to detect and prevent disease. But this philosophy and method is not accepted in modern medicine paradigms. We cannot casually reference the classical interpretation of tumors from the *Nei Jing* when discussing a case with an oncologist. Fortunately, at least half the didactic coursework for licensed acupuncturists is biomedicine. Medical terminology, anatomy, physiology, physical exam, lab analysis, red flag/emergency cases are all included in the curriculum to an almost equal measure. This means, we have an unseen advantage because of this comprehensive training. TCM doctors review and interpret pathology, physiology, and allopathic treatments

---

[21] MSKCC, 2018

and then (sometimes immediately) shift these findings into Chinese medicine concepts to create an individual treatment plan. Essentially, simultaneously translating from one medical language to another.

While this process can be straightforward for the common cold, when it comes to cancer, nothing is easy. Communication is imperative among providers of different training with equal regard for education, skill and expertise despite these known differences. Perhaps the acupuncturist at MD Anderson is accurate, and this duality assumes that the TCM profession is responsible for dialoguing with collaborative medical partners because we speak both languages. If that is what it takes, then ultimately the onus is on Chinese medicine doctors to introduce our medical vernacular as a valuable construct into the conversation with our IO colleagues. This is certainly the end goal. Until that time, however, the significant obstacles that create barriers to integration must be recognized and averted.

Dr. Di Giulio had the unique privilege to intern at a prominent IO facility during her doctoral program. It provided an opportunity to observe IO model of care and the promise of a collaborative healthcare network. What became most evident was the routine logistical barriers imposed on the Chinese medicine practitioners that overshadowed the healthcare team's potential for collaboration. The Cancer Treatment Centers of America (CTCA) in Tulsa, Oklahoma is a well-established cancer hospital. This is a reputable facility, which was founded in the late 1980s by Richard J. Stephenson who envisioned a cancer center with comprehensive medical oncology. Disillusioned by the treatment his mother received during her cancer diagnosis, he developed a multidisciplinary facility with all services under one roof. The philosophy of patient-empowerment and patient-centered care is embedded in the CTCA mission. It is appropriately referred to as the "Mother Standard" of care.

CTCA is considered a destination hospital. Every step of treatment from initial consultation to imaging, labs, chemotherapy, radiation, surgery and extended stays occurs onsite. This is appealing for patients and caregivers who can rely on complete supervision and quick access to medical care. Conventional medicine is the cornerstone of treatment at CTCA, but complementary therapies are numerous and extensively available. Physical therapy, cold-laser therapy, nutritional counseling, mind-body services, pastoral care, naturopathy, and acupuncture are on the menu of services.

There is also entertainment and activities, such as bingo, movie nights, daily exercise groups and transportation to events in the community. This exemplifies an approach that considers psychosocial wellness, quality of life, and acknowledges the needs of the patients beyond biomedical parameters of care.

At CTCA, acupuncturists fall under the umbrella of "Naturopathic Therapies." This department is led by a naturopathic physician and is comprised of licensed acupuncturists, naturopathic residents and doctors, most of whom are dual-trained in acupuncture therapy as well. This influences the structure of the department accordingly. In the hierarchy of this particular component of complementary medicine, naturopathy comes first and then Chinese. As such, the disconnect among the disciplines is apparent. Furthering this divisiveness was the fact that naturopaths shared offices in one area of the hospital while Chinese medicine was in another. Paths only crossed in corridors and hallways unless there were meetings. Communication about shared patients occurred by way of electronic charts. Thus, there were clear indications that the separate scopes of practice remained precisely that, separate.

A more integrative collaboration appeared in a process called grand rounds. Oncologists, nurses, social workers, therapists, pastors and naturopathic doctors (ND) are invited to attend and check-in with their shared patients. At the time of this internship, the licensed acupuncturists were not included in these collaborative rounds. The understanding was that the naturopaths represented the department. This process illustrated a significant discrepancy in the ideology of IO. In this example, there are two distinct features. Firstly, naturopathic medicine is an entirely different discipline, compared to TCM, not better or worse. It is likely more respected because of its scientific methodology as an evidence-based medicine, which better aligns with the West. Secondly, this particular environment results in minimal regard for TCM, which inherently implies that acupuncture is simply a technical modality. The clinical observations showed just that: short intakes, needles in, needles out, and repeat. The practitioners were very busy and stated they were strongly encouraged to treat even more patients per day. Considering the demands, the acupuncturists remained focused and provided immeasurable concern, compassion and care for their patients.

Similar to the other IO hospitals researched, neither moxibustion or Chinese herbal medicine was permitted. A request for an air filter or secluded space for moxa was denied. The reasons included available space and according to the acupuncturist who made the request, moxibustion was not science-based and was therefore not a proven, useful modality to integrate. Despite a conversation with a medical oncologist who condoned Chinese herbs and made attempts to introduce them on-site, he was met with skepticism and concern by colleagues and administration. Thus, basic herbal therapy was recommended by naturopaths and only what was available for purchase at the pharmacy.

The most distinctive feature of this internship reflected the aspect of "the language of medicine." In a small meeting led by an ND, attended by one acupuncturist, medical oncologist and research analyst, the idea of a scientific study on the merits of a particular acupuncture protocol for a pain-related condition was discussed. The first impression of this subject matter was encouraging. This discussion was a true picture of integration, and an opportunity to create a clinical study that warrants acupuncture for a particular condition as a result of cancer treatment. The barrier was evident within moments. The ND and medical oncologist were merely focused on the point combinations based on their individual indications to treat the pain syndrome. In an attempt to contribute and describe the theory and principles of TCM, the acupuncturist explained that there is more depth to be measured. Diagnosis, pattern differentiation, tongue, pulse — all of these elements contribute to the selection of acupuncture points to treat any condition. Protocols cannot be haphazardly applied without considering the constitution supported by the current presentation. This would essentially compromise the efficacy of the study.

The information was not met with a willingness to understand, and communication quickly faltered. There was no open discussion that considered alternative approaches for the study. The meeting ended abruptly with no resolution. While this is just a mere moment and glimpse into an honest attempt at integrative partnership, it appeared to reflect the larger issue of the IO paradigm. Conventional medicine along with disciplines that are scientifically affiliated and evidence-based, to a significant extent, control how complementary therapies, such as TCM, are accessed and studied. The range of application is grossly limited, relying upon a singular pillar to do all the work. This contradicts the nature of integration. It not only diminishes the capacity to build upon medical skills, but it also limits the ability to embed them into new paradigms, and most importantly, to heal patients.

The internship at CTCA was invaluable on many counts. It created a tangible, visual overview of an IO hospital that emphasized compassionate cancer care. While the components of integration were lacking, there was a genuine intention to that end. Following this experience, the doctoral research continued, and the investigation for the nebulous definition of integrative oncology went on. However, it became apparent that the concept and its application were indeed left up to interpretation. This was illustrated in a meta-analysis survey study performed by the Journal of the National Cancer Institute (JNCI). The conducted research reviewed 20 extensive definitions of IO. Predominant themes revolved around concepts of evidence-based medicine, management of symptoms, improving quality of life and complementary medicine in conjunction with conventional methods.

The compilation of terms and defining characteristics of IO overlap extensively. They are ingredients to a larger recipe, some parts unique and other elements predictable. Nonetheless, these formed a grouping that allowed deeper analysis toward a unified definition. The following statements are examples discovered by JNCI that highlight the varied components that encompass this growing specialty. Statements include:[22]

> "Integrative oncology is the term being increasingly adopted to embrace complementary and alternative medicine (CAM), but integrated with conventional cancer treatment as opposed to being considered a rival or true 'alternative'."

> "In the United States, the term 'integrative oncology' may be variably defined, but most definitions would include the idea and practice of adding complementary and alternative medicine (CAM) approaches to the range of therapeutic options provided to cancer patients in previously strictly conventional medical environments."

---

[22] Witt, 2017

> "…comprehensive, evidence-based approach to cancer care
> that address all participants at all levels of their being and
> experience."

This definition adapts current notions of "integrative medicine" — the judicious integration of CAM and conventional therapies in the best interest of patient — to oncology, with emphasis on aspects of patient care including attention to "body, mind, soul and spirit within the self, and within the specific culture and the natural world."[23]

The analysis of 20 definitions identifies characteristics, philosophies and themes that reflect a cohesive whole. With deliberation, a reliable foundation emerges upon which the definition is clearly derived in order to delineate clear guidelines within this specialty. Of the entire list, the shortest quote in length and description, stood out as a simple, approachable, all-encompassing framework, "Integrative oncology aims to combine the best practices of conventional and complementary oncological therapy (the 'best of both worlds')."[24] Indeed, it is often the remarkable features and strengths that an individual entity can bring that contribute to a greater whole. Equal balance optimizes better integration.

However, simplicity is not well received in the field of oncology. This has been demonstrated for hundreds of years as doctors, researchers, scientists, patients and caregivers strive toward a cure. It is evident that this nefarious disease demands complex, innovative treatments that eradicate the cancer cells and not the whole organism. To this end, the agreed upon definition of integrative oncology, finally unveiled in 2017 at the international conference led by SIO, reflects this inherent complexity:[25]

> "Integrative oncology is a patient-centered, evidence-informed
> field of cancer care that utilizes mind and body practices, natural products, and/or lifestyle modifications from different traditions alongside conventional cancer treatments. Integrative
> oncology aims to optimize health, quality of life, and clinical
> outcomes across the cancer care continuum and to empower

---

[23] Balneaves, 2018
[24] Witt, 2017
[25] Balneaves, 2018

people to prevent cancer and become active participants before, during, and beyond cancer treatment."

When we encountered this long-awaited definition, it was encouraging. It references mind-body medicine and natural therapies that occur in conjunction with allopathic methods. But, closer examination reveals the concept and ideology grossly differ from the practical application evident in analyses of IO facilities. It exemplifies a harmonious balance among disciplines, that does not easily exist. This suggests that practitioners of all backgrounds, skills and education collaborate alongside one another without a medical hierarchy. However, current systems do not reflect these standards. This standard of integration is inherently compromised by a myriad of logistical challenges, impaired by differing therapeutic views and practices, and then further hindered by an inability to communicate in one medical language.

The definition is a starting point, but it is not the ultimate guide. A window of opportunity is open to establish proper integrative dynamics that recognize the value of each medical modality. This fluidity aligns with the nature of the disease itself. As it evolves, so too must the providers and patients. Within that construct, there is an ebb and flow of interpretive understanding and from this evolution, improved application. This is what we aim to do by exploring the therapeutic capacity of traditional Chinese medicine for cancer. Peering beyond the romanticized version of acupuncture therapy and demonstrating the refined approaches and inherent value of this ancient medicine.

References

Abrams, D. I., & Weil, A. (2009). *Integrative Oncology*. New York, NY: Oxford University Press.

Balneaves, L. (2018). President's Message. *SIO NewsWire August 2018*, 1–2.

Kaptchuk, T. J. (2008). *The Web That Has No Weaver: Understanding Chinese Medicine*. New York, NY: McGraw-Hill.

MD Anderson Cancer Center. (2018). *Acupuncture*. Retrieved September, 7, 2018, from MD Anderson Cancer Center: https://www.mdanderson.org/patients-family/diagnosis-treatment/care-centers-clinics/integrative-medi-cine-center/clinical-services.html

MD Anderson Cancer Center. (2018). *Integrative Medicine Program*. Retrieved October 1, 2018, from MD Anderson Cancer Center: https://www.mdanderson.org/research/departments-labs-institutes/programs-centers/integrative-medicine-program.html

Memorial Sloan Kettering Cancer Center. (2018). *Developing Your Personal Care Plan*. Retrieved September 14, 2018, from https://www.mskcc.org/cancer-care/diagnosis-treatment/symptom-management/integrative-medicine/expertise

Memorial Sloan Kettering Cancer Center. (2018). *Individual Therapies*. Retrieved October 18, 2018, from https://www.mskcc.org/cancer-care/diagnosis-treatment/symptom-management/integrative-medicine/therapies/individual-therapies Video

Reddy, B. (2018). Acupuncture in an Integrative Oncology Center. *Acupuncture Today*.

Sagar, S. (2008). The integrative oncology supplement: A paradigm for both patient care and communication. *Current Oncology*, 166–167.

Seely, D., & Young, S. (2012). A Systematic Review of Integrative Oncology Programs. Retrieved September 10, 2018, from http://www.current-oncology.com/index.php/oncology/article/view/1182/1078

Witt, C., Balneaves, L., Cardoso, M., *et al.* (2017). *Comprehensive Definition for Integrative Oncology* | JNCI Monographs | Oxford Academic. Retrieved October 14, 2018, from https://academic.oup.com/jncimono/article/2017/52/lgx012/4617827

2 History of Oncology through Western and Chinese Medicine

"All things change, and we change with them."

Chinese Proverb

Despite cancer's persistent and dominant presence in medicine today, its roots extend back thousands of years. This long history exemplifies the disease's complex and resilient nature. Cancer has not been discriminatory through its course of medical evolution; just as the early societies of the West endured cancer's pervasive character for thousands of years, so did the East. While the title of oncologist did not emerge until the late 1900s, the mention of benign and malignant tumors appears across ancient medical texts. Early physicians across the world were discovering the intricacies of this pervasive disease, many with similar theories to its roots. Although now the biomedical dynamics of cancer in modern medicine are well understood, it is important to explore the historical evolution of this aggressive illness to understand the power behind it.

The timeline of cancer begins quite early with evidence of cancerous cells existing in fossilized dinosaur bones approximately 80 million years ago.[26] In 3000 B.C., Egyptian mummies were found to have cancer in fossilized bone as well, suggestive of osteosarcoma or bone metastasis.[27] The first written record of cancer is from 1550 B.C. where descriptions of surgical procedures on tumors were illustrated on Ebers Papyrus, one of the

---

[26] Cancer Council Victoria, 2013
[27] American Cancer Society, 2018

oldest preserved Egyptian medical documents. [28] Within the 110 pages of the scroll, there are 700 remedies and formulas to address numerous health conditions. Specifically related to cancer, the scroll cites eight references to tumors on the breast. It was believed cancer was an illness caused by the gods. It's described as a virulent disease, recounting "a tumor against the god Xenus" it recommends, "do thou nothing there against."[29] Essentially stating that there was no remedy for cancer. It may be assumed that even in 1600 B.C. cancer was a powerful entity of unknown origin treated with uncertainty and poor outcome.

The Ebers Papyrus describes treatment of these tumors with a heated instrument called "the fire drill," which was a form of cauterization to excise the cancer; the inscriptions suggest that treatment of this disease was only palliative. Other references to surgical procedures for ulcers and tumors are noted by "cutting out with a knife or burning with red-hot irons," which also describes the excision of tumors through surgical means.[30] From 500–1500 A.D. similar procedures were employed mainly surgery and cautery for smaller tumors; pastes containing arsenic were applied to the skin as well for more severe cancers; phlebotomy (blood-letting), and references to powder of crab as well as magical/symbolic charms were used. Herbal and nutritional remedy was also an integral component to ancient medicine with certain recommendations for cancer. Medical manuscripts describe stomach cancer treated with boiled barley mixed with dates; uterine cancer was treated with a blend of pig's brain mixed with fresh dates and inserted into the vagina.

In ancient China, the word, cancer (ai), itself was not referenced specifically until 1171, where it was stated in a text written by Dongxuan Jushi, entitled Wei Ji Bao Shu [A Treasury of Relief and Treatment]. Preceding this reference, there exists a long history of observation and treatment of tumors noted in classic medical texts. As early as the Shang Dynasty (16th–11th century B.C.), there is evidence found on bones and tortoise shells from where the word for tumor, liu, is identified.[31] In the Qin Dynasty (221–207 B.C.), physicians documented their observations of tumors, sores, suppurations, as well as theories on the disease. There was, of course, no

---

[28] Links, 1995
[29] Cancer Council Victoria, 2013
[30] ibid
[31] Peiwen, 2003

specialty for oncology during the early dynasties of the East. However, in the Qin Dynasty, doctors were classified with specialties such as internal disease, dietitians, and specialists of sores or wounds. Doctors of the latter condition treated sores with and without ulceration, termed "swollen sores." Traditionally, tumors were not divided as benign or malignant, but rather, according to visual and palpable characteristics.

A remarkable observation discussed in ancient dictionaries from the early 2nd century of the Han Dynasty (206 B.C.–220 A.D.), *Shuo Wen Jie Zi* (Discussing Characters and Explaining Words) and *Zheng Zi Tong* (A Comprehensive Discussion on the Correct Use of Characters) also delineates the difference between *zhong* (swelling) and *liu* (tumor). An abscess that is swollen and ulcerating is described as *zhong*, and *liu* equates to its homophone meaning, "to flow." Thus, the stagnation of *qi* and blood causes a swelling, or tumor: *zhong liu*. It is further explained that *liu* does not grow with the tissue but is rather the result of extended, chronic disease. It is remarkable that this concept is still applicable today and well understood in TCM diagnosis in two ways. First, the accumulation of *qi* and blood causes stagnation; and second, this accumulation may lead to acute or chronic disease, including cancer. In total, the diagnosis of *qi* and blood stagnation results from proliferation of tissue, inflammation and essentially, lack of flow.

In the West, a word for cancer, *karkinos* was first noted in medical literature during the time of Hippocrates.[32] Hippocrates (460–370 B.C.), recognized as the "Father of Medicine," is largely responsible for naming the disease. He noted that the structure of a tumor with its swellings, blood vessels and suppurations resembled a crab in the sand with legs spread in a circular fashion. This imagery influenced physicians, patients, and others affected by the disease who described the pain of cancer as being similar to the pain of being caught in a crab's pincers; or the physical quality of a hard, matted tumor, resembling the shell of the crab body; and how the movement of a crab reflected the fluidity of a tumor's growth under the skin.

Hippocrates' initial analysis of the disease is remarkable given the lack of technology, microscopes, scientific method, or knowledge of basic cellular division. His awareness of *karkinos* was quite limited and specific to

---

[32] Mukherjee, 2010

visible cancerous formations, such as breast tumors or skin cancers. Further, there was no way to differentiate malignant from benign, and many physical maladies fell under the umbrella of *karkinos*: general swellings, polyps, pustules, nodes and glands. Despite this limited scientific evidence and understanding of the disease, Hippocrates noted the aggressive nature of the disease, stating cancer was "best left untreated, since patients live longer that way."[33]

Hippocrates theorized the cause of disease as a result of an imbalance among four humors, or body fluids: blood, phlegm, yellow and black bile.[34] This is referred to as humoral theory, the first of many theories on the biology of cancer. When in excess, black bile was deemed to be the culprit of cancer, and this theory was accepted as the cause for over 1,300 years. Black bile was associated with *melancholia*, the medieval word for depression, and it was thought that this particular fluid congealed in the area where tumors formed. This theory is remarkably similar to those of the ancient Chinese physicians regarding stagnation of phlegm pathologies.

Five centuries later, a famous Greek physician, Claudius Galen, furthered Hippocrates' humoral theory through his medical observations. Galen also differentiated disease by excess of body fluids, some of which are realistic metaphors of modern day medicine, such as his understanding of inflammation as red, hot, with distending pain as a result of excess blood.[35] Jaundice was perceived as a result of excess yellow bile and is now commonly associated with production and function of the liver; and pustules, tubercles and nodules of lymph that were often white and cool in temperature, reflected excess of phlegm. These conjectures maintain threads of similarity and truth in current medical diagnosis for liver disease or infections and viruses.

Hippocrates and Galen both determined of the four humors, black bile was most dangerous. It was believed one's emotional health was inextricably linked with physical wellness within the scope of cancer pathology. Galen proposed that black bile was "trapped" cancer stating, "Of blacke cholor [bile], without boyling cometh cancer."[36] Galenic theory identified

---

[33] Mukherjee, 2010
[34] Sudhakar, 2009
[35] Mukherjee, 2010
[36] ibid

cancer as a systemic problem due to an excess of black bile, which created outcroppings of tumors throughout the body. Galen surmised removing tumors surgically was impossible because of black bile being deeply internal and throughout the body. Surgeons could attempt to excise a tumor, but the body would put forth more black bile immediately, so surgery was not advised.

Galen primarily attempted treatment of cancer by systemic means to eradicate the black bile. Remedies for cancer included lead tinctures, arsenic extracts, fox lungs, boar's tooth, ipecac and senna to name a few.[37] Pain was controlled with alcohol and opium tinctures. Rarely did Galen perform surgery, but some evidence suggests he did for palliative or cosmetic reasons. If the internal medical treatment was not effective, the most common method for treating cancer was a series of bleeding and purging techniques to literally extract the humors out of the body. This particular approach is an interesting comparison to an acupuncture technique used to resolve excess blood stagnation or heat referred to as bloodletting. Galen and Hippocrates' early theorizing and attempt to understand the nature of cancer play an inherent role in the biology of cancer setting a foundation for the medical advances that followed.

Similar to Western physicians, Chinese doctors were making early attempts to identify tumors and treat them effectively. The *Huang Di Nei Jing [The Yellow Emperor's Internal Classic]* is a core text of Chinese medicine; TCM would not exist without this comprehensive manuscript. In this classical literature, there are numerous descriptions of cancer-like formations, one may ascertain that the described masses, superficial sores or swollen areas of tissue could have been identified as early cancers. For example, early references to tumors include *chang liu*, identified as intestinal tumor and, *xie ge*, masses below the diaphragm due to blood stasis, and *ge sai*, an obstruction within the diaphragm.[38] The translations elucidate the type of mass, location and quality. *Shi jia*, is described as stone-like masses in the uterus. In modern medicine this could be diagnosed as ovarian cysts, fibroids, or gynecological tumor.

The *Nei Jing* created a foundation for developing theories related to etiology of tumors. The fundamental basis of Chinese medicine diagnosis is

---

[37] Mukherjee, 2010
[38] Peiwen, 2003

rooted in aspects of excess and deficiency, and the factors that play a role in this delicate dynamic are pertinent to good health. This is specifically discussed in the *Nei Jing* where emotions such as joy or anger may result in the accumulation of pathology, which may linger and cause imbalance.[39] It also states that environmental influences such as seasons that are excessively warm or cold, may perpetuate illness. Interestingly, in modern medicine there is recognition of environmental toxins and external influences that are linked to cancer formation. Also, significant to this assessment is the proper movement of *ying qi* (nutritive *qi*) and *wei qi* (defensive *qi*), both integral to upholding a strong immune system.

Tumor pathology is referenced throughout Qin and Han dynasties (221 B.C.–220 A.D.) and within classical texts such as the *Nei Jing*. Not only are the symptoms of the condition depicted, but also more importantly, they formulate TCM theory in order to understand the pathogenesis of the disease. For example, in the *Nei Jing*, in reference to intestinal *tan*, the famous physician Qi Bo states, "Pathogenic Cold settles outside the Intestines and struggles with *Wei Qi* (Defensive *Qi*). *Qi* cannot be nourished and will stagnate so that masses will form in the interior, pathogenic *Qi* will be aroused and polyps produced."[40] This answer by Qi Bo suggests a pathogenic factor (like one of the six excesses) will lodge interiorly and effect proper movement of *qi* and blood. As a result, there is an accumulation of these substances that provide opportunity for disease to manifest, such as cancer. Further, if the person's constitution is already deficient, the capacity of the pathogen to overtake what remains of the individual's health becomes even more harmful.

The Chinese classics note that pathogens can invade deeply when there is a constitutional deficiency. This concept is reflected in the *Ling Shu*, Chapter 75, which is essentially saying that pathogens or "evils" in TCM, particularly cold and heat, but also wind and fire, will invade into the interior when there is deficiency. A constitutional deficiency allows for a deeper and perhaps more tenacious penetration of an evil. The evil struggles with the defensive *qi* and the *qi* and/or fluids around it eventually trapping them and forming knots. These knots become tumors. At first soft, they grow as they

---

[39] Peiwen, 2003
[40] ibid

linger and become more dense and more recalcitrant. If the evil strikes into or at the level of the sinews, then a sinew tumor is formed, and if into the intestines, then an intestinal tumor is formed, and so on.[41] These diagnostic elements to TCM theory are extremely important in clinical medicine. The practitioner must identify the constitutional deficiency and assess the strength of pathogenic factor with respect to the subject's constitution in order to effectively treat with acupuncture and herbal therapy.

A more detailed analysis of the theories presented in the *Nei Jing* takes place in the *Nan Jing (Classic on Medical Problems)*. This is where pattern differentiation evolves specifically pertaining to oncological theory and development in Chinese medicine. The description of benign versus malignant tumors is discussed in the 55th Problem stating, "Accumulations consist of *yin* influences...stay in the depth and are hidden...emerge in the five depots... Their upper and lower extensions are clearly marked by end and beginning; to the left and to the right are clearly defined locations where they subside."[42] The *Nan Jing* also states that illness that arises in the depots (*zang* organs) are difficult to cure. That is a patient is likely to die. In contrast, an illness that arises in the palaces (*fu* organs) can be difficult but is easy to cure. That means that a patient should live. This accumulation mass, related to *yin* and a disorder of the *zang* organs (five depots) has the same qualities of what is now perceived as a malignant tumor given the structure, definitive location and shape. By contrast, a concentration is described as being a problem with the *fu* organs (six palaces), thus related to *yang*, not maintaining a specific area or shape. In a clinical perspective, the concentrations were most likely assumed to be benign, perhaps that of a lipoma or fibroid. In essence, ancient TCM doctors could already classify cancer as a disease that affected the whole system, not merely limited to external causes. Further, one's internal constitution and overall health determined, to some extent, the absolute strength of pathogenic factor.

Back in the West, by 1540, a physician named Andreas Vesalius unknowingly challenged the humoral theory made by Hippocrates. This occurred through Vesalius' dedication to understanding human anatomy

---

[41] Unschuld, 2016
[42] Unschuld, 1986

by way of autopsy on human cadavers, something Hippocrates was unable to perform for religious reasons during the Grecian era. Through detailed anatomical research Vesalius determined that the black bile referenced by Hippocrates and Galen did not physically exist.[43] Through autopsy he discovered the pale, watery fluid of the lymphatic system, the blood vessels holding blood, and the liver holding yellow bile.[44] Black bile was not found, which challenged Vesalius not only on a professional and academic level, but also on a personal level through his dedication to his predecessor, Galen. In his search, without realizing the outcome, he produced extensive diagrams of veins, nerve pathways, and the circulatory system, culminating in the first medical anatomy book, *The Seven Books on the Structure of the Human Body*. As a result, the humoral theory was cast aside and physicians began to search for another source of cancer, which lead to the lymph theory.

Lymph theory proposed that the cancer formation was caused by another body fluid, lymph. This idea was supported largely through the 17th century and suggested that the human body was formed of lymph, which was responsible for the ongoing movement of blood and fluids. Blood released tumors into the body's circulatory system, eventually leading to cancer in that local region. Not long after this theory was introduced, the evolution of cancer biology made significant progression in the medical field with the discovery of cellular biology. As scientists could examine cellular structure in closer detail, it became evident that cancer is actually made up of cells derived from other cells. Thus, the observed character of the disease continued to become more illuminated, as science, technology, and physicians identified its mechanism.

This cellular discovery led to the blastema theory, developed by pathologist Johannes Muller in 1838 who recognized the cellular com-position of cancer.[45] He proposed that cancer was cellular and not lymph fluid believing further that cancer cells were a separate entity from normal healthy cells. His student, Rudolf Virchow, became one of the foremost

---

[43] British Broadcasting Channel, 2014

[44] Mukherjee, 2010

[45] American Cancer Society, 2014

leaders in pathology. His scientific research led to the understanding that entire organisms do not get sick, but it is the cells or groups of cells within the organism that do.[46] Thus, cancer cells did not originate from body fluid but from other cells. Virchow played a significant role by initiating the field of cellular pathology following the advent of the microscope. As such, Virchow revolutionized the field based on two tenets: first, similar to the bodies of animals and plants, human bodies were made up of cells and second, cells arise from other cells.[47]

This greatly influenced the practice of medicine as physicians began to recognize that disease progression occurred by pathological and anatomical changes not merely as a result of symptom changes. Physicians could then make more effective medical diagnoses and treatments, ideally with better outcomes. The similarity of animal's anatomical structures shed light on the pathology and physiology of humans, which was the advent of harnessing animal research into human biology and medicine. Virchow proposed a hypothesis about the distinction of cellular human growth, which differentiated between hyperplasia and hypertrophy. Virchow defined the primary method of cell change, hyperplasia, as a growth of cells increasing in number, versus hypertrophy, where the number of cells did not change, but rather individual cells grew in size. It's possible to delineate the structure of human tissue by hypertrophy and hyperplasia. For adult animals, fat and muscle grow through hypertrophy. By contrast, internal organ structures such as the liver, intestinal tract, blood and integumentary system all grow through hyperplasia.

As a result of Virchow's knowledge and studies on cellular pathology, he proposed cancer was a result of pathological hyperplasia. With a microscope, Virchow examined abnormal cellular progression, identifying a significant aspect of uncontrolled cellular growth — hyperplasia. The structure of cancerous cells appeared more clearly through this process allowing a distinct point of view. Essentially, cellular division occurred autonomously in a different, new form; hence the term, *neoplasia*, "novel, inexplicable, distorted growth."[48] As a consequence, these cells

---

[46] Schultz, 2008
[47] Mukherjee, 2010
[48] Ibid

expanded into dense masses, invading normal tissue with the drive to metastasize to surrounding organs and other distant sites such as the brain, bones or spinal cord.

By the 19th century, the complexity of cancer was gaining momentum in the scientific community. The biology and evolution of the disease were more clearly delineated by scientists Watson and Crick who discovered the deoxyribonucleic acid (DNA) helical structure in 1953 and subsequently received the Nobel Prize in 1962. Following this discovery, geneticists were able to identify how genes worked, as well as how they were damaged by mutations causing cellular division. Encompassing this discovery was the integral component of carcinogens, like chemicals affecting DNA structure, as well as changes in cellular integrity by viruses, radiation, or genetics.

In 1970, the discovery of two gene families provided even more information on cancer cell biology. Proto-oncogenes are normally responsible for controlling the frequency to which a cell divides, and the degree to which it differentiates. When these genes mutate uncontrollably or abnormally, they become malignant, and an oncogene is created. Oncogenes are not always activated or turned on, but when triggered, it may lead to neoplasm. Tumor suppressor genes were also identified. Normally these genes control cell division, the repair of damaged DNA and instruct cells when to die off. If the tumor suppressor gene does not function, this impairs the control of cells causing overgrowth and division. Both oncogenes and tumor suppressor genes are negatively impacted by chemical exposure and radiation. In addition to these groups of specific gene families, scientists also found genetic predispositions to cancers such as those that affect the thyroid, pancreas, colon, kidney and ovary.

As modern medicine evolved, so did the ability to treat cancer more effectively, as illustrated by the various methods employed by oncologists today. The current treatment of cancer has fortunately extended beyond "the fire drill" procedure from ancient Egypt, to more modern and mainstream treatments like surgery, chemotherapy and radiation. The early administration of conventional medicine was far from flawless, requiring numerous attempts and many years to refine techniques in cancer care.

TIMELINE:	WEST:	EAST:
80 million years ago	Cancerous cells found in fossilized dinosaur bones	
3000 B.C.	Egyptian mummies were found to have cancer in fossilized bone	
1600 B.C. to 1501 B.C.		**Shang Dynasty**: evidence found on bones and tortoise shells, where the word for tumor, *liu*, is identified
475–221 B.C.		**Warring States period**: *Huang Di Nei Jing* includes descriptions of cancer-like formations
460–370 B.C.	A word for cancer, *karkinos* was first noted in medical literature.	Tumor pathology is referenced in classic medical texts that formulate TCM theory of the disease
221–207 B.C.	Hippocrates develops **four humors theory**, an imbalance among the four humors: blood, phlegm, yellow and black bile	**Qin Dynasty**: Physicians documented their observations of tumors, sores, suppurations and theories on the disease
206 B.C. – 220 A.D.		**Early Han Dynasty**: *Shuo Wen Jie Zi* and *Zheng Zi Tong*, early dictionaries, delineate the difference between *zhong* (swelling) and *liu* (tumor), equating to benign and malignant **Late Han Dynasty**: *Nan Jing* describes pattern differentiation, specifically pertaining to oncological theory
1171		**Jin Dynasty**: Initial reference to cancer (*ai*) by Dongxuan Jushi, entitled *Wei Ji Bao Shu* [A Treasury of Relief and Treatment]
1600s	**Lymph theory** develops, cancer formation was caused by another body fluid, lymph	
1838	**Blastema theory**, cellular biology is developed, cancer is actually made up of cells, derived from other cells	
1900s	The complexity of cancer gains momentum in the scientific community.	

Allopathic Forms of Cancer Treatment

Surgery

Surgical removal of tumors was the first form of cancer treatment. In ancient medical approaches to cancer, physicians recognized that cancer would likely return even after surgery.[49] Due to limitations of sanitary surgical procedures, as well as proper tools and anesthesia, surgery was risky and complicated. There were higher rates of blood loss and often death. Once anesthesia was developed in 1846, surgeons were able to perform more complex surgeries to remove tumors. This era was referred to as the "century of the surgeon."

The physician commonly identified with oncological surgery is Dr. William Halsted, a surgeon in the late 19th century. He is regarded as the doctor most responsible for developing the radical mastectomy. His assertion was that cancer could be eradicated through local removal of the tumor and surrounding tissue, which began with the removal of the pectoralis minor, then extended into the chest, collarbone, surrounding lymph nodes, anterior mediastinum, and for his disciples, there are records of removing ribs, amputating a shoulder and collarbone.[50] He determined, if there was a reoccurrence, it was due to a new neoplastic disease process and not related to the primary cancer that was eradicated. This radical mastectomy became the foundation for cancer surgery in the century that followed, until the 1970s, when surgeons were able to modify the mastectomy using more sophisticated techniques and making it less disfiguring with fewer side effects.[51]

During this same time period (late 19th – early 20th century) another physician, Stephen Paget, determined that cancer cells could spread from the primary tumor through the bloodstream to another location in the body.[52] This unique and significant concept was eventually proven in modern day medical research because of technological advances that explain cellular biology and the process of metastasis. As Paget's findings became

---

[49] American Cancer Society, 2014
[50] Mukherjee, 2010
[51] WebMD, 2014
[52] American Cancer Society, 2014

more readily acknowledged in the medical community, physicians recognized the limitations of cancer surgery, in that, full excision of a tumor and the surrounding area did not equate with a curative outcome. In addition, systemic treatments after surgery were developed to enhance the rate of survival by continuing to destroy malignant cells; this also lessened the extent to which surgery was performed, thereby decreasing the surgical mutilation. Exploratory surgery was often required to make a complete diagnosis of cancer, but with the advances of ultrasound and imaging, invasive surgeries are quite limited. This has occurred due to the development of chemotherapy and radiation, both of which have a more recent history and continue to be a mainstream approach to combating a cancer diagnosis.

Radiation therapy

Radiation therapy, also known as radiation oncology or radiotherapy was discovered after the advent of the X-ray. In 1896, a German physics professor by the name of Wilhem Conrad Roentgen presented a lecture entitled "Concerning A New Kind of Ray" and within months, the scientific community had designed systemic approaches and X-ray machines for identifying broken bones or locating foreign objects.[53] Further research on the element radium proved quite successful, as scientists found that radium also killed diseased cells, targeting damaged DNA. There began a new and instrumental era of medical oncology.

Currently, at least half of all cancer patients are prescribed some form of radiation therapy.[54] Scientific advancements in the field of radiation therapy have improved greatly. The precision of radiotherapy has been refined to offset unnecessary exposures. There are several methods of radiation therapy, which include: proton beam therapy (targets tumor cells directly), stereotactic surgery and therapy (gamma knife used for brain tumor), and intra-operative radiation therapy (applied after surgical removal of tumor to adjacent tissue). These advanced surgical techniques have allowed oncologists to truly refine their practice, thus providing patients with enhanced quality of life and potential for better outcomes.

---

[53] American Cancer Society, 2012
[54] Krans, 2017

Chemotherapy

About the same time that radiation therapy was discovered in the early 1900s, a German chemist by the name of Paul Ehrlich began developing drugs to treat illnesses.[55] The concept of chemotherapy as systemic medicine came from this research, and the term *chemotherapy* was born defined as the use of chemicals to treat disease. It appeared to be a natural progression to use chemical compositions in order to create a drug for the treatment of cancer. However, the evolution of chemotherapy agents has been constantly challenged by the concept of specificity. Specificity refers to a medicine's ability to differentiate between its intended target and its host. "The trouble lies in finding a selective poison, a drug that will kill cancer without annihilating the patient. Systemic therapy without specificity is an indiscriminate bomb."[56]

It wasn't until World War II, when researchers observed United States Navy sailors who were exposed to mustard gas during military activity and who experienced changes in bone marrow cells. As a result, scientists began to examine nitrogen mustard and its effects on white blood cells in the bloodstream or bone marrow when dosed in a controlled setting. After animal studies confirmed that malignant cells in blood and bone marrow disappeared without the negative effects of nitrogen mustard, doctors prescribed the chemical agent on humans with lymphoma. Almost immediately, swollen glands decreased in size, and it appeared as though remission was inevitable. Unfortunately, relapses were imminent and patients' tumors would grow, harden, and the cancer would return. Nonetheless, nitrogen mustard inspired scientists and chemotherapists to continue research on chemical agents that might effectively destroy rapidly growing cancer cells by damaging their DNA.

In 1954, The National Cancer Institute (NCI) was authorized by the Senate to create cancer research-based programs. This led to the development of the Cancer Chemotherapy National Service Center (CCNSC), which allowed scientists to test chemotherapeutic drugs in controlled targeted settings. From 1954–1964, over 82,000 synthetic chemicals were tested,

---

[55] Devita & Chu, 2008
[56] Mukherjee, 2010

including 115,000 fermented products and 17,200 plant derivatives.[57] The significant amount of research on chemical formulations reflected the fervent hope of finding curative substances for cancer. However, the decades that followed included many challenges for the chemotherapist.

Medical oncology was not a designated specialty in the 1960s. Those who administered chemotherapy were not regarded as specialists of cancer, but rather, referred to with less reputable names. For example, Louis K. Albert, who was involved in initial studies on nitrogen mustard and early lymphoma cases was known as "Louis the Hawk and his poisons" simply because he was often present during chemotherapy infusions. Quite simply, anti-cancer drugs in the 1960s were predominantly considered to be poison and not medicine. This sentiment has not completely disappeared in modern day cancer treatment.

Nonetheless, research continued and was led by those with utmost commitment to finding a cure for cancer through effective safe chemotherapy. The discovery of aminopterin, a compound related to folic acid, proved successful through its ability to promote remission in children with Acute Lymphoblastic Leukemia (ALL). This drug was the predecessor of methotrexate, one of the oldest chemotherapy drugs frequently used in treatment today. The evolution of chemotherapy continued rapidly and by the 1970s, adjuvant chemotherapy was introduced. Adjuvant chemotherapy is employed after surgery to kill any micrometastatic disease that may remain, thus preventing a recurrence. This is similar to the approach of administering radiation post-operatively to lessen the degree of growth for small tumors unable to be surgically removed.

By 1971 the "war on cancer" had formally begun as a result of the National Cancer Act. This act instituted a substantial amount of funding, which allocated billions of dollars for research specific to drug development and clinical trials. The momentum from this increase in funding escalated research in cancer pathology and more refined chemotherapy treatments. Additional systemic treatments were extrapolated including hormone therapies, targeted therapies, immunotherapies and biologic therapies. These categories of drugs would not exist without the dedication and courage of early oncologists who participated in the

---

[57] Murherjee, 2010

advancement of chemotherapy. From the mid 19th century to present day, this research has been integral to the development of successful, therapeutic outcomes in a cancer diagnosis.

Timeline:	Treatment:
Pre-19th century	Surgical removal of tumors was the first form of cancer treatment
19th century	"Century of Surgery" Early 19th century: term *chemotherapy* was born
1846	Anesthesia was developed
1896	Radiation oncology or radiotherapy discovered after the advent of the X-ray
1954–1964	National Cancer Institute (NCI) authorized by the Senate to create cancer research-based programs; leads scientists to test chemotherapeutic drugs in controlled targeted settings
1960s	Medical oncology becomes designated specialty
1970s	The "war on cancer" declared; surgery becomes more refined; adjuvant chemotherapy introduced

The history and evolution of Chinese medical oncology proceeds without much deviation from its historical findings. The classical references to tumors date back over 2,000 years, and astonishingly, the theoretical applications remain the same. Chinese medicine's methods of *zang-fu* pattern differentiation, as well as addressing the individual's constitution, were aspects to oncology evolution that were not included in the Western medical paradigm. In current practice, Chinese medicine continues to adhere to the foundations of diagnosis through examination of the following: *zang-fu, yin-yang* theory, five elements, meridians and collaterals, *qi* and blood, body fluid, six excesses and five emotions. Within TCM, a continuity exists. The diagnostic methods are based on principles that reflect nature; these principles evolve with nature as they were intended to do. In modern day China, the practice of TCM and Western medicine, which was brought in during the 1900s Cultural Revolution as a means to modernize the country, are blended as a hybrid model of medicine.

It is evident through its historical evolution, that the aggressive nature of cancer has existed for thousands of years. Although it persists, statistics indicate that there is a downward trend of the disease with overall improved outcomes. It requires a certain hypervigilance by those who choose to practice in the field of oncology, and even more so by individuals diagnosed with cancer.

References

American Cancer Society. (2012). *Evolution of Cancer Treatments: Radiation*. Retrieved November 3, 2014, from American Cancer Society: http://www.cancer.org/cancer/cancerbasics/thehistoryofcancer/the-history-of-cancer-cancer-treatment-radiation

American Cancer Society. (2014). *Evolution of Cancer Treatments: Surgery*. Retrieved September 7, 2014, from www. cancer.org: http://www.cancer.org/cancer/cancerbasics/thehistoryofcancer/the-history-of-cancer-cancer-treatment-surgery

American Cancer Society. (2014). *Early theories about cancer*. Retrieved October 31, 2014, from American Cancer Society: http://www.cancer.org/cancer/cancerbasics/thehistoryofcancer/the-history-of-cancer-cancer-causes-theories-throughout-history

American Cancer Society. (2018). *Early History of Cancer*. Retrieved October 14, 2018, from https://www.cancer.org/cancer/cancer-basics/history-of-cancer/what-is-cancer.html

British Broadcasting Channel. (2014). *History: Andreas Vesalius*. Retrieved September 8, 2014, from bbc.co.uk: http://www.bbc.co.uk/history/historic_figures/vesalius_andreas.shtml

Cancer Council Victoria. (2013). *Cancer Council Victoria*. Retrieved September 14, 2014, from Cancer Council Victoria: www. cancervic.org

Devita, V. T., & Chu, E. (2008). *A History of Cancer Chemotherapy*. Retrieved November 3, 2014, from Cancer Research: http://cancerres.aacrjournals.org/content/68/21/8643.long

Krans, B. (2017). Radiation Therapy. Retrieved August 29, 2018, from https://www.healthline.com/health/radiation-therapy

Links, C. (1995). http://www.crystalinks.com/egyptmedicine.html. Retrieved August 7, 2014, from Crystalinks: www.crystalinks.com

Mukherjee, S. (2010). *The Emperor of All Maladies*. New York, NY: Scribner.

Peiwen, L. (2003). *Management of Cancer with Chinese Medicine*. St. Albans, Herts, UK: Donica Publishing Ltd.

Schultz, M. (2008). *Rudolf Virchow*. Retrieved September 7, 2014, from National Institute of Health: http://www.ncbi.nlm.nih.gov/pmc/articles/PMC2603088/#!po=10.0000

Sudhakar, A. (2009). *History of Cancer, Ancient and Modern Treatment Methods.* Retrieved September 7, 2014, from National Institute of Health: http://www.ncbi.nlm.nih.gov/pmc/article/PMC2927383/

Unschuld, P. U. Trans (1986). *Nan-Ching, The Classic of Difficult Issues.* Berkeley: University of California Press.

Unschuld, P. U. (2016). *Huang Di Nei Jing Ling Shu — the ancient classic on needle therapy.* Oakland, CA: University of California Press.

WebMD. (2014). *Radical Mastectomy for Breast Cancer.* Retrieved September 7, 2014, from Webmd.com: http://www.webmd.com/breast-cancer/radical-mastectomy

3 Chinese Medicine Diagnosis and Acupuncture

"Medical theories can not be explained to those who are superstitious with ghost or gods; and the magic effect of acupuncture will not be acknowledged by those who do not believe or dislike acupuncture. Those who do nor allow treatment of a disease will certainly not be cured, and treatment by force never has good results."

Neijing

It is difficult to write about any modality of TCM, especially acupuncture, without including a discussion on diagnosis. For a treatment to be complete, the pillars that comprise the medicine depend on one another and become inseparable, like *yin* and *yang* itself. Therapeutic outcomes rely upon a formulated diagnosis, which in turn informs the methodology of each modality. The result is a formulated treatment plan that promotes the pillars to function synergistically in alignment with the diagnosis. In essence, acupuncture, moxibustion, herbal prescription, manual therapy, nutrition and exercise are integral components built upon the foundation of diagnostic assessment. For example, trained Chinese medicine physicians do not begin a treatment with acupuncture without determining the underlying root condition and branch presentation. The aspect of diagnosis is so crucial that it could easily necessitate a book of its own, and fortunately, there are classical texts and modern scholars who have contributed to the principles, patterns and theories that continue to evolve Chinese medicine oncology diagnosis. This groundwork serves as a clinical launching pad that enables an already competent starting point in TCM oncology treatments.

The intent of this chapter is to enhance diagnostic and treatment approaches whether a student of Oriental medicine or new practitioner interested in integrative cancer care. For the seasoned clinician, these principles may seem elementary. The acupuncture points associated with diagnostic patterns will be familiar to TCM doctors. And yet, recognizing the synergy of these points according to the location of a tumor, stage of disease or patient symptom is extremely relevant and can never be perfect. Thus, the goal of this chapter and subsequent acupuncture therapy techniques is to make the overwhelming intricacies of neoplastic disease clear and more accessible. The material does not cover the wide array of cancers and the extensive angles of treatment. We leave that to the skill of the practitioner, where again we see the inherent aspect of art versus science. Through this lens, the following information is intended to broaden the scope of acupuncture therapy techniques in private practice and as part of integrative oncology programs.

This chapter is dual-focused. First, it is an introduction to Chinese medicine's diagnostic patterns associated with stages of cancer. These principles are extrapolated from specialists in TCM oncology who agree upon the primary elements of the pathology and development of tumors. Second, from this vantage point, the focus shifts into practical applications of acupuncture therapy. Here, the scope broadens from the simplistic form of point indication and treatment of symptoms for acute, palliative care and instead leans into therapies that access the whole organism, mind and body. Our experience in integrative oncology showed that acupuncture was primarily used for symptom management, but it has far-reaching effects when practitioners think outside the box.

Further, the inherent value of diagnosis is part of a continuum in Chinese medicine. So, while this section covers acupuncture therapy for cancer management, the core diagnoses can be applied in the subsequent chapters that review moxibustion, herbal medicine or nutrition. It is important to note that just as there exist many schools of thought in the treatment of disease in Chinese medicine, TCM oncology is an evolving, complex specialty with a multitude of approaches. The unifying thread among these practices is the formulation of a diagnosis. Regardless of which medical background one ascribes to, whether allopathic or traditional, the common theme in cancer management, is that there is no straightforward diagnosis, treatment or cure. Thus, integration of diagnoses ultimately benefits the cancer patient by providing whole person medicine in order to improve outcomes, the true nature of integrative oncology.

In Western culture, acupuncture tends to be the most well-known and widely accepted modality of TCM. Many people erroneously consider acupuncture to be the entirety of Chinese medicine perhaps because it is the most heavily scrutinized by Western medical researchers. It has been argued that historically acupuncture played a relatively minor role in TCM treatment, comprising roughly 15% of the medicine. Despite critique from traditional science-based medical paradigms, it has been upheld as a valuable form of complementary medicine. Thus, acupuncture is frequently misrepresented as the primary tool of the trade. Integrative oncology promotes its usage primarily for palliative care purposes to alleviate cancer-related symptoms. An unfortunate byproduct of this current trend is the tendency to carve acupuncture into a technical pathway that disregards theory, principles and diagnosis.

The function of acupuncture therapy is to create balance and regulation through a combination of points that correspond to a specific diagnosis and treatment principle. In the myriad stages of cancer, there is an intricate array of treatments that correlate to the principle pattern, type of cancer, location and stage of the disease. Within this context, it is important to distinguish the primary diagnosis from the numerous side-effects of the cancer itself. There is often an interplay of both the disease and its effects, a continuous cycle that calls for attention due to the nature of the illness, and its response to conventional medicine. In addition, TCM pattern differentiations include a subdivision of distinct diagnoses for each type of cancer. This means there is always multifactorial presentations and complex patterns with excess and deficient symptomatology. The treatment principle is established based on a number of aspects such as underlying constitution, age, gender, lifestyle, environmental exposures, as well as etiology and pathology.

It is common for modern practitioners to simply translate a Western diagnosis in TCM terminology or put too much emphasis on the acute, symptomatic aspects of the patient's condition. This is evident in various "acupuncture protocols" in cancer management, a concept that inherently contradicts the methodology of Chinese medicine. These interpretations dismiss the distinct manner of diagnostic assessment. Oncologists would not prescribe chemotherapy without a definitive cancer diagnosis. So, why would practitioners of TCM practice acupuncture without the same sort of definitive diagnosis? And yet, there are an increasing amount of trainings for licensed acupuncturists, some even led by medical doctors with a certification in acupuncture, that have developed point protocols to treat side-effects and cancer-related conditions, a practice that disregards diagnostic assessment. This is evident by the referrals we receive from oncologists that indicate specific requests to alleviate symptoms and side effects, such as nausea and vomiting, fatigue, and pain with acupuncture.

This oversimplification is illustrated by two features: symptom and point indication. For example, PC-6 (*nei guan*) is commonly used for nausea and vomiting, making it indispensable for cancer patients experiencing these symptoms likely due to cytotoxic therapy. It is an effective point for gastrointestinal discomfort caused by the chemotherapeutic agents that injure the middle *jiao*. However, it is necessary to determine the cofactors of diagnosis to inform treatment principle and point selection. Much like the concept of the pre-existing condition familiar to Western healthcare, Chinese medicine considers the patient's constitutional patterns that may indicate causative factors. For example, is there a history of Spleen *qi* deficiency or internal cold that damaged the Spleen *yang*? If the patient is elderly, how prominent is the Kidney deficiency? Are there emotional stagnations that impair the Liver and cause it to overact on the Spleen and Stomach? These queries better inform the practitioner, who can then formulate a TCM diagnosis to selectively combine supportive points with PC-6 (*nei guan*) for a more therapeutic treatment.

The Chinese medicine patterns that accompany a cancer diagnosis are multifaceted. The disease impairs the physiological body alongside injuries caused by conventional treatments. These inter-related variables shift rapidly during active cancer, which demands close attention to diagnostic strategy. More importantly, these strategies must seamlessly integrate with advanced biomedical concepts and interventions. Modern literature on the subject of Chinese medical oncology demonstrate that TCM scholars agreed upon the etiology of tumors. These patterns include excess pathologies, specifically: *qi* stagnation and blood stasis, damp phlegm accumulations, and binding of toxic heat. Deficient causative factors relate to *zang-fu* weakness of channels and organs, as well as body substances, like blood, *yin* and *yang*. These defined principles led to distinct perspectives and approaches on how to best treat malignancies, which considers more than just the cellular pathology.

TCM treatment strategies are devised by placing equal value in the assessment of the patient's constitution, relative to the stage and severity of the neoplasm. Within these tenets, the most integral principle in cancer treatment with Chinese medicine, embedded in cancer management, is the concept of *Fu Zheng* therapy, which is to always supplement the root or vital *qi*. As Western medicine is successful in targeting tumors and controlling cancerous spread, it subsequently damages the internal terrain of the body, weakening the immune system and the body's ability to fight disease. This is when *Fu Zheng* therapeutics are uniquely suited as an integrative modality.

Core diagnostic and treatment principles of traditional Chinese medicine and cancer:[58]

- Early (I-II) stage: The tumor is localized with no degree of spread, and the patient's health and constitution are strong. Therapeutic strategies focus on eliminating the excess pathogens, clearing heat and toxicity, tonifying the vital *qi* and supplementing the root.
- Intermediate (II-III) stage: The tumor has spread beyond the site of origin to adjacent tissues or lymph nodes, but the patient's overall health remains stable. The treatment strategy aims equally to dispel the pathogenic factors and to clear heat toxicity, as well as to strengthen vital *qi* and to nourish the root.
- Late (III-IV) stage: Metastatic spread has occurred and cancer cells have invaded other organs and areas of the body causing weakness and debilitation. The primary strategy is first to nourish vital *qi* and to tonify deficiencies. This is followed by dispelling pathogenic factors.[59]

This outline presents a diagnostic guideline that bridges biomedicine with Chinese medicine principles at each stage of neoplastic disease. It reflects the inherent concept of balance and regards the whole person

---

[58] Peiwen, 2003
[59] ibid

from disease to the energy of the physical-emotional body. Of note, each stage tonifies vital *qi* and strengthens the root, but the weight of this focus shifts according to pathology and patient health. We have observed TCM clinicians who focus overwhelmingly on dispelling the excess pathology, such as toxic heat or blood stagnation, without considering the patient's capacity to respond to such a treatment. For example, in a diagnosis of stage IV breast cancer with metastatic spread, the patient is likely depleted after extensive rounds of chemotherapy or conventional treatments. This injures the *qi* and *yin* of the body, which further diminishes as the excess pathogenic factors (heat toxin, phlegm and blood stasis) overwhelm the constitution. Regardless of the extent of spread and the pathogenic influences at hand, the appropriate treatment strategy necessitates a greater ratio of tonification compared to reduction methods.

This makes sense for a couple reasons. To begin with, the abnormal division of cells that precedes a cancer diagnosis is in a sense, opportunistic. Meaning, the environment of the body is compromised to some degree, which can be considered a relative weakness or an opportunity for illness. Second, while it is possible for an excess pathogen to overcome the defenses of a strong and healthy person, the modern-day lifestyle of "work hard, play hard" and never really "turning off" becomes a dangerous dynamic. This cycle lends to deficient patterns, indirectly generating excess pathologies that are essentially rooted in deficiency. Third, allopathic medicine injures the body in its effort to eradicate cancer cells. This method is equivalent to the TCM principle of dispelling or draining toxicity, but Chinese medicine has the added advantage of strengthening the whole person to optimize the healing response according to a root and branch system of diagnosis.

Excess Etiologies

Etiological factors that generate excess pathology in the disease of cancer are multifactorial. This concept parallels the discussion on TCM diagnosis in that it demonstrates the importance of evaluating the patient's core constitution relative to the cancer itself. These patterns can be distinguished individually but must also be examined in partnership with integration of Eastern philosophy and Western medicine. Through this perspective, the excess patterns that occur in relation to cancer are compared to the West's biomedical framework. These diagnoses include *qi* stagnation and blood stasis, damp and phlegm accumulations, and toxic heat syndromes.

Qi Stagnation and Blood Stasis

One of the predominant excess conditions in the disease of cancer is stagnant *qi* and blood stasis. This presentation is merely one component to the progression of cancer. Its pattern can be identified as a precursor to the disease, as this congestion inhibits healthy circulation of blood in the body. Left untreated in a state of imbalance and immobility, stasis can perpetuate the formation of masses or tumors. A classic image of this concept involves a boat in the water. If there is enough water (*qi*), the boat floats and is moved by the current (blood). If there is not enough water, or it is stagnant, the boat becomes stuck. By comparison, Western medicine views blood as a fluid that can be placed under the microscope. So, it is well understood as a tangible substance that shares an inordinate amount of information about the cellular health of the patient. The TCM concept of blood stasis correlates to the literal components of blood, such as the role of platelets and clotting factors. Obstructed blood is visible in varicose veins, broken capillaries, or bruising. These are identifying factors of obstructed blood that perpetuate deeper disharmonies that lead to disease. (Refer to Table x.)

The Integrative Lens of *Qi* Stagnation and Blood Stasis: Eastern vs. Western

TCM	Western
Sharp, stabbing pain	Platelet aggregation, clotting factors
Worse with pressure	Blood coagulation
Tongue: dark or purple	Bruising, varicose veins, broken capillaries
Pulse: choppy	

Interestingly, Chinese medicine has the capacity to observe signs of internal stasis even before a patient is aware of them. The diagnostic methods of tongue and pulse examination can indicate imbalances that signal specific treatment approaches that promote blood circulation and tonify *qi* in order to mobilize it. The tongue may be purple with sublingual veins, and the classic quality of the pulse is choppy. The phases of stasis evolve over time and can occur from a variety of factors that include acute or chronic injury, poor diet (inflammation leading to stagnation), a lack of exercise, and/or suppressing emotions, to name a few. Often it is not until a patient complains of persistent discomfort or notices a swelling or mass that medical attention is sought. By this time, the pathology is well-established and a condition such as cancer requires the reactive approach of conventional medicine. But if stasis is identified early on, then the method becomes one of preventing disease before it happens instead of after.

Classic qualities of *qi* and blood stasis include pain that is fixed, stabbing, worse with pressure, improved by movement and unrelieved by rest. It is important to distinguish if one factor is greater than the other in order to focus treatment. Sometimes stuck *qi* is more predominant than *blood* or vice versa. Also, determining the overall strength of the *qi* is of equal importance. Deficient *qi* must be strengthened in order to promote circulation. Treatment principles inform the combination of acupuncture points and modalities utilized to address the diagnosis of *qi* stagnation and blood stasis.

The primary meridians provide numerous points to facilitate the movement of *qi*, invigorate blood and dissolve blood stasis. The following list of points are common examples indicated for promoting circulation: SP-6 (*san yin jiao*), SP-10 (*xue hai*), LV-3 (*tai chong*), LV-14 (*qi men*), UB-40 (*wei zhong*), LI-11 (*qu chi*), LU-5 (*chi ze*), UB-17 (*ge shu*). Other considerations include *xi-cleft* points along the channel to address acute pain and *ashi* points, or areas of tenderness adjacent to or distant from the tumor site. Beyond these customary point selections, there are unique systems and acupuncture techniques that treat stasis patterns.

For example, pricking therapy on the *jing-well* point of the affected channel releases blood stagnation to reduce pain and to clear inflammation. This is a basic starting point for bloodletting therapy most TCM students learn in school. But there is a vast range of potential in this technique, which we have readily adopted into our clinical practice. Modern interpretations and clinical applications must be credited to Chinese medicine doctor, Henry McCann, whose recent book *Pricking the Vessels*, outlines this intricate system and technique. His exposition on Master Tung's map of the body indicates specific zones that correlate to an anatomical area. Bloodletting techniques of the indicated zone is an effective method to promote microcirculation and eliminate stasis as an indirect form of treatment.

This method was applied routinely for a 38-year-old male patient with stage III stomach cancer. The "Stomach zone" is located on the dorsal aspect of the feet surrounding ST-41 (*jie xi*) and traverses toward the toes. Indications include stomach cancer, abdominal pain, gastric ulcers, hiatal hernia.[60] Inspection and palpation of the region may identify variations in skin texture or areas of redness, distended veins or capillaries, which all indicate stagnation and warrant pricking technique. Preceding his cancer diagnosis, the patient complained of a constant burning and heavy, sharp pain in his epigastrium that worsened over a period of months. He attributed these symptoms to stress and adjusted his diet. The discomfort did not resolve, and there was no relief from antacids recommended by his doctor. A gastroenterologist ordered an endoscopy, which identified a tumor with metastatic spread to his lower esophagus. This stasis expressed as a result of underlying Spleen deficiency and emotional constraint that influenced the Liver to overact on the middle *jiao*. This degree of internal stasis is just one aspect within the continuum of tumor pathology in Chinese medicine.

For this patient, pricking the "Stomach zone" was a regular part of acupuncture treatment as supportive therapy to eliminate the internal stasis, alleviate pain, clear heat and move blood. Before the chemotherapy regimen began, analysis of the Stomach zone revealed purple, distended veins within the area, a diagnostic sign of internal *qi* and blood stasis. During chemotherapy, imaging scans confirmed the tumors decreased in size. Interestingly, alongside this outcome, assessment of the Stomach zone indicated a lighter color overall with less distension and dark capillaries. In essence, this observation paralleled the success of the cytotoxic therapy that decreased the size of tumor (*qi* and blood stasis). In each TCM treatment, the Stomach zone was evaluated to determine the relative degree of stagnation in his epigastrium and became an integral component to his cancer management with Chinese medicine. This demonstrates the manner in which medical disciplines, despite different diagnostics and treatments, can integrate methods to promote medical outcomes.

---

[60] McCann, 2013

Pain is frequently reported in patients with malignant tumors due to size and location of a tumor may impinge nerves, surrounding tissue or organs causing discomfort. For example, a 60-year-old, non-smoking female presented in our clinic with what she initially thought was an orthopedic complaint. She had reported the symptoms to her doctor, describing severe upper body pain that affected the right shoulder, scapula and upper arm for several weeks that increased in frequency and intensity. There was limited range of motion and significant discomfort upon palpation. Her doctor prescribed a course of physical therapy, but it did not work. She continued to suffer until a magnetic resonance imaging (MRI) was ordered, which showed a large mass extending from the thoracic vertebrae to the shoulder capsule. Pathology confirmed stage IV nonsquamous cell lung cancer. In TCM principles, this late-stage diagnosis reflects substantial *qi* and blood stasis, evident by the extent of the mass itself. Moreover, underlying patterns of Liver *qi* stagnation with damp accumulation, and Kidney-Lung *yin* deficiency were apparent. Thus, the physical expression of dysregulated *qi* and blood is evident, but its etiology is a pathogenic blend of injuries.

General point prescriptions include primary meridians along the affected channel that reduce pain and local inflammation. They function to facilitate movement of *qi* and promote circulation, such as: UB-18 (*gan shu*), PC-6 (*nei guan*), LI-4 (*he gu*), UB-40 (*wei zhong*), LV-3 (*tai chong*), GB-34 (*yang ling quan*), Du-20 (*bai wei*), and *ashi* points. The inherent function of points can serve to dissolve the tumor by virtue of their ability to mobilize and disperse accumulations. Biomedically, studies have shown needling points with these indications will increase metabolic activity locally, while preventing platelet aggregation and tumor growth by promoting fibrinolysis.[61] While classic meridian theory is an invaluable source for modern practitioners, Chinese medicine encompasses a wide range of acupuncture therapy systems, for example, the eight extraordinary meridians (EEM).

The *Chong* is uniquely suited to address patterns of *qi* and blood stasis with acute or chronic pain syndromes. Its inherent characteristic of both holding and disseminating blood systemically means that it carries great capacity to resolve local areas of congestion. The *Chong* associates with the source *qi* of the Kidneys and connects with the *San Jiao* channel, which

---

[61] Peiwen, 2003

is responsible for the movement of this energy. In the case of the patient above with lung cancer, the *Chong* was incorporated into her treatment plan with dual function and purpose. First, to treat the widespread obstruction of *qi* and blood that caused intense, acute pain levels. The *Chong*'s link to the *San Jiao* facilitates movement of stuck *qi* that disperses accumulation, which in turn decreases discomfort. Second, the combination of injury due to the disease characteristics, as well as the harsh and aggressive radiation protocols further depleted her *qi* and Kidney *yin*. Therefore, the *Chong*'s relationship to the Kidney strengthened this physiological aspect to tonify, to generate more energy and to rebuild a stronger foundation.

Damp and Phlegm Accumulations

A challenge in the scope of integrative oncology is to distinguish the pathogenic characteristics among more esoteric systems, such as TCM, in relation to the scientific structure of Western medicine. This is particularly true for TCM doctors who observe the innate workings of the body in manners that cannot be easily translated or measured by the standards of evidence-based disciplines. A close exception to the rule is within the context of damp-phlegm accumulations, which has some overlap with the West's literal concept of phlegm. This pathology can be interpreted as a substance with tactile properties: a congealing fluid that is sticky, mucus-like, white, yellow or green in color. It is one of the easiest terms to explain to patients because of these shared characteristics that are easy to visualize. Therefore, in consultation with patients who are curious about the nature of Chinese medicine and how it perceives a disease like cancer, there is an opportunity to use the concept of phlegm to further elaborate.

Part of the explanation can provide an overview of the role of damp-phlegm in tumor growth, but masses and tumors are actually congealed formations of stasis: *qi*, blood, phlegm and often toxic-heat. Tumors are analyzed with biomedical diagnostics from the moment they are discovered. This process refers to staging of the cancer. Several components are necessary to determine the extent of the disease. This includes a complete physical examination with careful palpation of the area of concern that assesses the skin and lymph nodes. Further analysis occurs through surgery to locate, measure and resect the tumor, if possible. Pathology reports examine the cancerous tissue that further lead to a definitive diagnosis. These findings are compiled into a complete picture of the disease profile from which a treatment plan and prognosis is made. It is summarized into a clear staging system that TCM providers must be familiar with: TNM. This refers first to the magnitude of the tumor (T), lymph node involvement (N) and metastatic disease (M).

The biomedical findings are extremely useful for the TCM physician, who can interpret these results into our own principles and theory of disease. The size, location and extent of the tumor in the body is an instrumental aspect in considering the degree of damp, phlegm, stasis and/or heat. This excess pathology can be compared to underlying deficiencies. We observe TCM practitioners glancing over lab reports, who would greatly benefit from a more comprehensive understanding of conventional strategies like staging, which is an unfortunate reality in the spectrum of current integrative practice approaches. The formation of a tumor, as an acute manifestation is directly linked to the constitution and lifestyle of the patient, which must be considered in order to effectively treat in conjunction with Western oncological protocols.

As referenced, tumors and masses are accumulations of damp or phlegm. The substantial forms of phlegm are classified as being a thick, turbid, congealing fluid. Excess pathogenic factors are derived from internal deficiency or external influences, such as heat invasion that causes a fever, or a strong wind invasion that triggers a common cold. Damp is part of the group of external pathogens that easily invades the body. Thus, if the external source is profoundly robust, it can override the body's response and illness presents. By contrast, if the person is immune-compromised, or relatively weak, then the internal deficiencies create an open terrain for pathogens to enter, such as damp.

The deficiency associated with damp-phlegm accumulation is primarily linked to the health of the Spleen and Kidney meridians. A weakened Spleen, perhaps as a result of poor diet, cold foods, overwork or worry, sets the stage for damp invasion or internally generated dampness. Conversely, long term presence of dampness, such as obesity, inhibits the function of the Spleen, and its ability to generate healthy *qi*. This is a common clinical presentation when patients complain of fatigue and inability to lose weight. The Kidney's role in metabolizing water and fluids can be further impaired by damp. This failure of normal fluids to be transformed and transported through proper channels will create dampness, which will lead to stagnation. This stasis of damp or phlegm may generate cold or heat and this combination is conducive to neoplastic growth, particularly if there is constitutional weakness.

Draining damp is a classic TCM principle that corresponds to this presentation. Needling points that transform phlegm, soften hardness and dissolve lumps are extremely beneficial with tumor formations of any size. Cofactors of heat, *qi* and blood stasis may be present, but the emphasis on expelling damp is crucial to stimulate movement of the static area. Points indicated for damp conditions include: SP-9 (*yin ling quan*), SP-3 (*tai bai*), SP-4 (*gong sun*), LV-2 (*xing jian*), UB-20 (*pi shu*), KI-7 (*fu liu*), Ren-9 (*shui fen*). ST-40 (*feng long*) is used for sticky, turbid phlegm, which we incorporate with stage III-IV cancers with metastasis. Some practitioners like Dr. Li Peiwen approve needling around the mass or accumulation, in essence, *ashi* points.[62] Generally, we do not surround the tumor with needles even when it is visible and palpable. The tissue is already compromised and often sensitive from surgery or radiation. There simply is not enough information about the cellular response with local needling. In these cases, we refer to the Chinese medicine adage, "further takes you farther."

With respect to this philosophy, the *Ren* channel as part of the system of eight-extras therapeutically addresses damp-phlegm patterns. The *Ren* vessel traverses the midline of the body, beginning at the perineum, ending at the upper lip, where it meets the *Du* channel. By virtue of this course, its pathway connects to the pelvic region and corresponding organs. Tumors of the bladder, ovaries, uterus and lower intestine can be treated with the *Ren* meridian. In the theory of EEM, the *Ren* treats damp accumulations or internal obstructions, and symptoms such as vaginal discharge, swellings and masses. Its regulatory aspect of the endocrine system is particularly beneficial for hormone-related cancers. In cases with estrogen (ER) and progesterone (PR) positive breast cancers, the *Ren* promotes hormonal balance in its ability to nourish *yin* (akin to the West's understanding of estrogen) and regulate *qi*.

---

[62] Peiwen, 2003

Exposure to chemotherapy disrupts the normal rhythm of the menstrual cycle. In pre-menopausal women of child-bearing age, conventional treatments compromise the health of the ovaries. Measures to protect the reproductive system often include freezing eggs before they are injured, until treatment is complete, and the cycle regulates naturally. For peri- and post-menopausal women with ER/PR positive cancers, antiestrogen therapies are prescribed, such as Tamoxifen. These agents are used as disruptors that block the body's production of estrogen, in essence, cancer preventative.

In either clinical presentation, the dysregulation of hormones due to conventional treatments lead to significant imbalances of the physical and emotional body. There are symptoms that align with menopausal transitions, such as night sweats, hot flashes, anxiety, dryness and sleep disturbance. But, our clinical experience demonstrates that the emotional impact of diagnosis is almost as devastating as the physical impact. In these cases, we incorporate the *Ren* meridian because it is perfectly attuned to the mental-emotional aspects. Neediness, feeling disconnected, withdrawn, overcontrolling or being controlled in relationships and inability to connect are examples of more deeply-rooted patterns that tend to unfold and surface during cancer treatment. Thus, the versatility of the *Ren* treatment exemplifies an integrated strategy for hormone-related cancers as well as phlegm accumulations. While the West's strategy is effective in disrupting estrogen-related tumors, the East harnesses the natural regulation of *yin* for a healthy mental and physical hormonal terrain.

Heat Toxin

The third common diagnostic pattern that manifests in cancer is heat toxin. As an excess form, heat is considered a pathogenic factor that is derived from external or internal conditions. On its most basic level, heat develops through exterior invasions, much like contracting a flu that causes a fever. In other presentations, heat is generated internally from excess: *qi* and blood stasis, or by contrast: *qi* and blood deficiency. In both conditions, the lack of circulation increases the degree of heat, which becomes a conduit for further disharmony. If the body does not resolve the heat naturally, or if it is left untreated, it has the capacity to burn fluids (*yin*). Additionally, heat hardens phlegm accumulations engendering firm masses or tumors.

Fire is an escalation of latent heat patterns, which is to say untreated external pathogenic factors that align with modern infections or viruses. Taken one step further is heat toxin, classically associated with swift epidemics, such as malaria. Modern Chinese medicine considers the exposure of exogenous toxins in the environment as pathogenic factors that manifest as toxic heat syndromes, including cancer. Carcinogenic materials, synthetic chemicals, and countless ingredients in daily-life products have been identified as cancer-producing.

From this framework, the concept of heat toxin and its relation to neoplastic disease is apparent. While not always the case, this presentation occurs mainly with stage III-IV cancer. Heat toxin is a severe form of internal accumulation, which is less apt to happen in early-stage cancers. The micro-inflammation caused by tumors impairs the structural integrity of the adjacent blood vessels and tissues, which disrupts normal function. In essence, it impedes the smooth flow of *qi* and blood. When this regulation is missing, disease presentations escalate. Without sufficient blood supply, the inflammatory response controlled by the tumor causes further necrosis, ulceration and suppurative infection. These symptoms reflect the cofactors previously discussed: blood stasis and phlegm. The body's response to these presentations is a fever. Classic signs include: thirst, irritability, sweating and a surging, rapid pulse. More severe forms of heat toxin also may lead to mania, delirium and mental confusion. This excess pathogen also can stir the blood causing reckless bleeding. For example, tumors of the breast at late stages or left untreated can ulcerate superficially.

Acupuncture therapy is extremely beneficial for heat-related presentations because the actions of specific points clear heat, cool blood, drain damp and relieve toxicity. Common examples include: SP-10 (*xue hai*), LU-11 (*shao shang*), UB-40 (*wei zhong*), LI-11 (*qu chi*), Du-14 (*da zhui*), UB-22 (*san jiao shu*), GB-34 (*yang ling quan*), SP-9 (*yin ling* quan), LU-5 (*chi ze*), and SJ-5 (*wai guan*). *Ying*-spring and water points on the associated *yang* channel clear heat. For example, SI-2 (*qian gu*) is indicated for febrile diseases. LI-2 (*er jian*) is recommended in point protocols by integrative oncology hospitals to treat xerostomia, a common side-effect of chemotherapeutic agents. This reasoning correlates to its location on the channel as a *ying*-spring (clear heat) and water point (moistens). In addition, pricking therapy on the *jing-well* of the associated *zang-fu* is an effective needling method to efficiently clear heat and drain fire, as well as alleviate pain.

The interventions of Western biomedicine to eradicate tumor cells with surgery, cytotoxic therapy and radiation introduces further injury to the body. The intention is clear: rid the body of cancer. But the whole organism is compromised. Of these conventional methods, radiotherapy is the conduit for toxic heat invasion. When the physical body is exposed to radiation, it accumulates into toxic heat patterns that ultimately burn *yin* fluids. This in turn impairs the regulation of body fluids and causes dryness. Thus, the treatment principle is to moisten dryness, nourish *yin*, and clear heat toxins. Damage to the Spleen and Stomach effects the dynamic function of building blood, so points that harmonize these meridians are necessary. Examples of this point selection include: SP-6 (*san yin jiao*), Ren-6 (*qi hai*), LV-3 (*tai chong*), UB-18 (*gan shu*), UB-23 (*shen shu*), SI-2 (*qian gu*) and LI-11 (*qu chi*).

By comparison, the Liver and Kidney *yin* is equally injured by the toxic nature of chemotherapy. Deep nourishment of the Kidneys is integral to recovery. The *Chong* meridian, as an eight-extras treatment, accesses these components to care in its ability to connect with the Liver, Spleen and Kidney. The sequence of points begins with the opening point, SP-4 (*gong sun*). From there, the trajectory of point combinations is dependent on the patient's patterns and symptoms. The points we have incorporated during chemotherapy or radiation cycles, particularly in mid-late stage cancers with heat toxin pathology, consist of: ST-30 (*qi hong*), SP-12 (*chong men*), KI-16 (*huang shu*), KI-21 (*you men*), KI-27 (*shu fu*) and Ren-14 (*ju que*) or Ren-15 (*jin wei*). In addition to addressing the side effects, the Chong is deeply rooted in the true-self and reconnects the body and spirit.

Deficient Conditions

Compared to the diagnostic presentations of excess pathology in neoplastic disease, deficient patterns are less delineated but more prominent. At every stage of cancer, whether early or late, an element of deficiency is almost always identifiable. The degree of vacuity ranges in severity, as a response to the disease itself, and conventional medicine therapies. The mere presence of a tumor, however, means that deficiency is relative to the excess. The complex presentations that result are therefore a reflection of both the acute physiological response and constitutional factors. This intricate dynamic is expected in cancer management. An integral role of the TCM practitioner is to distinguish the root from the branch in the first clinical assessment to formulate principle patterns. The distinct aspects of a patient's lifestyle, such as tendency to overwork, stress levels, dietary and sleep habits indicate a great deal. Each answer is another piece to the diagnostic puzzle, which enables a more complete diagnosis.

In the West, there is widespread physical and emotional exhaustion. Chronic depletion disrupts the regulation and strength of the body. Over time this becomes a precursor to illness. In Chinese medicine, we examine these deficiencies very closely. Overwork injures the Kidney and Liver *yin* and causes vacuity, which in turn stagnates the Liver *qi*. This disharmony is at the root of many breast cancer pathologies. Women with a propensity for overwork become depleted over an extended period of time. The injury of the Liver *yin* and its subsequent stagnation, as well as its pathway through the breast are all causative factors in tumor formation. Liver stasis also overacts on the Heart in the Five Phases system. When there is Heart stasis, emotional disharmony occurs, such as insomnia and depression. Physical patterns include the possibility of accumulations or masses. Poor diet affects the Spleen's ability to transform and transport food and fluids. Overeating, high-fat diets, sugar and cold food or drinks inhibit the functions of the Spleen. This directly affects the Spleen *qi* and building of blood, leading to combined patterns of *qi* and blood deficiency.

The concept of deficiency in Chinese medicine is well-understood. Practitioners are trained to observe the nuances of *qi*, blood, *yin* or *yang* depletion patterns. Sometimes these are quite apparent in cases, but in most instances and certainly in the disease of cancer, a multitude of deficiencies are present and transform regularly. An established framework that outlines the stage of disease in relation to the concurrent deficiencies is a useful starting point in integrating treatments effectively. Through this structure of understanding, therapeutic principles guide clinical approaches that enhance outcomes and optimize the patient's response to the disease and Western medical interventions.

Qi and Blood Deficiency

The biomedical characteristics of early-stage cancer indicate a positive prognosis. The injury to the body is less severe because metastatic spread has not yet occurred. When the tumor is localized, total surgical resection is possible. This correlates with curable outcomes. When the disease remains in its tissue of origin and the patient's constitution is relatively strong, the primary treatment principle is to dispel the pathogenic factor (*qi*-blood stasis, damp-phlegm, toxic heat), followed by tonification of *qi* and concurrent *zang-fu* deficiencies. This establishes a formidable baseline that guides the therapeutic approach. Of equal importance is the consideration of constitutional factors relative to the excess pathology. For example, in an 80-year-old patient diagnosed with stage II stomach cancer, the treatment principle shifts in accordance with the patient's age and overall health. The primary focus is tonification of Vital *qi* and the Spleen and Kidney *yang* in order to strengthen the body and actively disperse the blood stasis pathology.

This occurs alongside the administration of chemotherapeutic agents and radiation that simultaneously disrupt the production of blood, from both a Western and Eastern viewpoint. The cytotoxic components of chemotherapy injure the bone marrow. This essential substance has delineated cellular structure that promotes circulation of mature blood cells throughout the body. Bone marrow is a tangible, spongy tissue deep within the bones responsible for the production of platelets and both red and white blood cells. This hematopoietic function generates leukocytes and granulocytes (neutrophils, eosinophils and basophils).[63] Each cell has a predetermined purpose in maintaining the health of the body. The cell's ability in oxygenation of tissue and protection from micro-organisms, encompassed by its own anatomy and life cycle, all play into the vitality of blood and solidifying it as a precious substance.

Consequently, blood is observed closely by Western and Eastern practitioners during conventional oncology regimens. A complete blood count (CBC) examines the red blood cells (RBC), white blood cells (WBC) and platelets. Patients are required to have a blood draw prior to a chemotherapy infusion to measure the status of this system due to injury of the bone

---

[63] Peiwin, 2003

marrow. Neutrophils are particularly subject to chemotherapeutic exposure causing a condition of neutropenia when counts fall below 1000/mm.[64] This deficiency predisposes the patient to bacterial infections. Neutropenia can escalate to neutropenic fevers, requiring antibiotics and delaying cyclical treatment. The nature of the febrile symptoms varies according to the individual. While some patients spike a fever rapidly, others experience low-grade intermittent fevers. Both require antibiotics, which in turn cause further injury to the gastrointestinal system and immune flora of the gut.

Chinese medicine equally reveres the substance and concept of blood. It is an aspect of *yin*, readily subject to injury through the combination of extensive treatments and the disease itself. Damage to the Spleen and Stomach disables the proper digestion of food and fluids. This directly impairs the body's production of blood. The symptomatology of stage I-II mimic classical signs of *qi* and blood deficiency. Interestingly, these correlate to neutropenic presentations: lethargy, low appetite, easily nauseated, dizziness and generalized weakness. Acupuncture therapy enhances the function of the Spleen to produce blood, which in turn supports the Kidneys in the production of marrow.

In both Western and Chinese medicine, marrow is an inherently valued substance. Its clinical characteristics are distinguished according to medical perspective. In Chinese medicine, marrow is considered one of the six extraordinary organs. The Kidney essence is the origin of marrow, which encompasses three distinct types of marrow: brain (Sea of Marrow), spinal and bone. Marrow is nourished by *jing* (essence) and controls intelligence, clarity and relates to the Heart blood and Liver. Thus, it nourishes blood, calms the spirit, promotes circulation of *qi* and regulates emotions. Chapter 33 of the *Ling Shu* states, "If the Sea of Marrow is abundant, vitality is good, the body feels light and agile, and the span of life will be long. If it is deficient there will be dizziness, tinnitus, blurred vision, fatigue, and a great desire to lie down."[65]

While it is rare to only incorporate acupuncture without supplementing with moxibustion or herbal medicine, there are instances in which acupuncture is the only option. In the following section we will focus on chemotherapy,

---

[64] Lahans, 2007
[65] Maciocia, 2005

above other Western interventions, to demonstrate how an integrated therapeutic approach coordinates with timed chemotherapy doses. This establishes a framework for the application of other TCM modalities that may be implemented alongside radiation or as pre-surgical support for example. This clinical method intends to improve the patient's response to the Western protocol throughout the cyclical phases of chemotherapy. It is more than merely palliative. Certainly, patients report a decrease in acute nausea, improved appetite and restful sleep. But more importantly, patients are able to complete chemotherapy rounds and radiation cycles without interruption, which is a primary goal in integrative cancer care.

In active chemotherapy cycles, it is common for patients to experience a fluctuation in energy patterns and acute symptoms. At its most basic, *qi* and blood deficiency underlie the continuum of pathology, but the degree of depletion is largely influenced by their constitutional cofactors to disease and biomedical regimen. This pertains to the cytotoxic agent, cycle duration and the nadir, all of which must be considered in the coordination of TCM treatments. There are numerous classifications of chemotherapy drugs based on specific actions. For example, platinum-based compounds are referred to as alkylating agents, such as cisplatin, which is commonly used in breast cancer protocols. Platinum-based chemotherapies are known to cause neuropathy as a predominant side effect. When we have the opportunity to treat patients before they begin chemotherapy protocol that include cisplatin, treatments can focus on preventing injury to the channels and *zang-fu* that are often affected.

In addition to knowing the associated side-effects of chemotherapy drugs, we also consider the nadir, which is the low point. In conventional medicine, it is a byproduct of chemotherapeutic treatments that reflects the lowest level of blood counts following an infusion. The irony of this relative low point is it occurs in between chemotherapy doses after patients have endured the most acute side-effects, which on average occur on the second and third day after an infusion. Once the nausea and vomiting resolve, energy rebounds and the patient reports feeling more like themselves. But this is likely when the nadir takes place. Therefore, acupuncture therapy that is timed according to the dosing schedule will preemptively decrease potential side-effects, and during nadir, rebuild *qi* and blood. For patients who are generally healthy (minor *qi* and blood *xu*) and the pathogenic factor (neoplastic disease) is relatively weak (stage I-II), we recommend the following Chinese medical approach to integrate with the conventional treatment accordingly:

Cycle Timing: Preceding Chemotherapy Infusion (day before or morning of)

Integrated Treatment Approach:
TCM: Tonify *qi* and blood, tonify Spleen, nourish Kidney, calm spirit
Western: Boost immunity and strengthen blood (WBC), alleviate emotional stress or nervousness

---

Channel Points: Ren-17 (*shan zhong*), GB-39 (*xuan zhong*), SP-10 (*xue hai*), LV-3 (*tai chong*), ST-36 (*zu san li*), Du-20 (*bai wei*), LV-13 (*zhang men*), KD-3 (*tai xi*), UB-23 (*shen shu*) *Yin Tang*

Master Tung: *San Cha San, Three Emperors: 77.17 (Tian Huang) or 77.18 (Shen Guan), 77.19 (Di Huang), 77.21 (Ren Huang)*

EEM: *Chong* and specific channel pathway to open the meridian that traverses the tumor, as well as connect to the patient's essence, and emotional healing. *Example: Stomach cancer and Ren*

Moxibustion: 3–5 cones on *Du-14* (*da zhui*) or GB-39 (*xuan zhong*)

Cycle Timing: Day 1–3

Integrated Treatment Approach: Strengthen *qi* and eliminate stasis, clear heat; alleviate and prevent cytotoxic side effects

Clinical note: Cycles of chemotherapy are infused with excess/deficient and cold/heat etiology. Pre-chemo steroids, anti-nausea, anti-anxiety and the chemotherapy regimen itself are cofactors in the patient's acute physiological response. Characteristics are unique to the case, but it is important to consider the properties of each medicinal compound relative to the patient's constitution and disease. Practitioners must become familiar with the chemotherapeutic agent, its expected side effects (acute and/or chronic), and nadir time period.

The following is a general list of acute side-effects commonly observed in clinic days 1–3: nausea, vomiting, low appetite, cancer-related fatigue, insomnia, night sweats, vivid dreams, constipation, abdominal pain and bloating, anxiety, fear, worry.

Primary Meridian Acupuncture: PC-6 (*nei guan*), LV-14 (*qi men*), ST-43 (*xian gu*), LI-11 (*qu chi*), LI-4 (*he gu*), SP-4 (*gong sun*), UB-20 (*pi shu*), UB-21 (*wei shu*)

Master Tung: *Shui Tong* (1010.19) and *Shui Jin* (1010.20)

Pricking Therapy: To address Spleen and Kidney deficiency with blood stasis (tumor), bloodletting of selected points on the *Yang Ming, Tai Yang,* or *Jue Yin* channels, which are replete with blood, is effective in reducing excess, pathogenic or latent heat, and clearing inflammation. In any disease differentiation, stasis must be lessened to encourage the production of fresh blood to nourish the Kidneys and essence.[66]

---

[66] McCann, 2014

Cycle Timing: Day 3–7 or Nadir
Clinical Note: Remember that on average, this specific time period following a chemotherapy infusion is when the patient feels more normal, but blood lab values are at their lowest. Our primary methodology during a patient's nadir is the moxa box (see Chapter 4) or other moxibustion techniques, but these can be supplemented with the following point recommendations.
Integrated Treatment Approach: Strongly tonify *qi* and blood, tonify *wei qi* to prevent illness or infection
Channel Points: Du-14 (*da zhui*), ST-36 (*zu san li*), LI-4 (*he gu*), SP-3 (*tai bai*), Ren-6 (*qi hai*), SP-6 (*san yin jiao*); UB-17 (*ge shu*) and UB-19 (*dan shu*), referred to as the Four Flowers is an excellent paired point combination for blood deficiency with blood stasis patterns. Classically, moxibustion is utilized. Clinical application of acupuncture on these points during nadir is effective in nourishing the depleted blood symptomatology, along with eliminating the stagnation (tumor).
Auricular: WBC support: Endocrine, Adrenal, Sympathetic, HT, LV, SP, KD;
Immunity: Spleen (Western and Eastern), Thymus, LU;
Anemia: Endocrine, HT, LV, SP, ST, Small Intestines
EEM: *Yin Wei:* Its energetic association with the pineal gland, which regulates melatonin for sleep, makes this channel therapeutic in its ability to promote restful sleep, allowing the body to replenish *qi* and blood overnight. Improved energy decreases risk of infection if exposed to colds or flus.
Du: Its inherent connection to *yang* energy facilitates deeper tonification of *qi* and *yang*, which influences the adrenals and immunity, as well as resistance to disease.

Blood and *Yin* Deficiency with Heat

In the advancement of neoplastic disease, we typically observe a progression from the presentation of *qi* and blood deficiency in stage I-II, to the development of more *yin* deficient conditions with heat. Unless the cancer was accelerated by an outside influence (excess pathogen), it is likely the cancer pathology has resided in the body for some time. The cellular tentacles have reached beyond the original tumor site to invade adjacent tissue and regions of the body. In Chinese medicine, long-term stagnation generates heat from the lack of movement, which can burn up the *yin* fluids of the body, like blood. Layer the harsh properties of chemotherapy or radiation that are infused into the body in forms of excess heat, alongside stagnation, then patterns of deficiency escalate. What begins as *qi* and blood deficiency triggers a sequence of depletion that eventually leads to *yin* deficiency, then *yin* deficiency with heat.

Stage II-III cancers are a comparative midpoint of disease. Clinically, patients diagnosed at these stages tend toward more apprehension and uncertainty. There is a distinct recognition that the disease was not caught early enough, and by comparison, are relieved it was discovered before an aggressive spread. Thus, the emotional energy is mixed. Aptly, so is the physical presentation. In these cases, the disease is more established at the blood level. More regions of the body are compromised, both anatomically and biomedically. The homeostasis of the *zang-fu* system is undermined by this imbalance, reflective in more pronounced physical manifestations with a higher ratio of deficiency compared to excess. This vacuity is intertwined with the formidable excess pathology, blood stasis and/or phlegm-damp accumulation.

The normal functions of the five *zang* (*yin*) organs and the six *fu* (*yang*) organs are impaired by a more developed neoplastic disease presentation as compared to stage I. Stage II-III indicates moderate level of spread. The measurement of the tumor is larger, and there is more concentrated spread into adjacent tissue, as well as lymph node involvement. This cellular process is an outcome of preexisting injury to the biological mechanisms of the body. Exposure to carcinogenic factors, partnered with improper diets, overwork and stress are all components to disease formation. This is not new information in even modern medicine standards. Chinese medicine views the ongoing depletion of the body's resources as intrinsic motivators toward chronic illness, such as cancer. Individuals who are not in tune to the messages from the internal body, essentially the warning signs of what's to come, will inch past stage 0-I cancer pathologies and into mid-late stage diagnoses.

Chinese medicine practitioners are familiar with these patient profiles. After extensive years observing cancer patients, we have had an opportunity to witness behaviors of so-called healthy patients that are clear warning signs. As the body ages and becomes more fatigued and less able to naturally dispel dampness, move *qi* fluidly and clear heat, early indicators of disease present. Often, these symptoms are mildly managed, largely ignored and patterns continue as if on auto-pilot. This concept is illustrated in the phrase "burning the candle at both ends," which Chinese medicine relates to Kidney *yin* deficiency. Cancer patients with stage II-III exhibit these signs. They were likely present before the tumor was identified, clearly evident through the diagnostic assessment and definitely by conventional methods of care.

The therapeutic approach for cancers diagnosed as stage II-III encompass the range of methods noted in the previous section for *qi* and blood deficiency. However, the clinical difference is the inclusion of more *yin* nourishing points, with greater focus on clearing excess and deficient heat. The angle of care adjusts to the terrain of mid-stage illness, which is more complex. It is a delicate balancing act of treatments that observe the continuum of pathological patterns, the disharmony of vital substances and how both interrelate to *zang-fu* deficiency. The treatment principle for this stage appropriately focuses on these therapeutic concepts, imparting more focus on enriching *yin* and moistening body fluids.

The role of acupuncture therapy for any stage of cancer is to facilitate the body's innate ability to heal and transforming disharmony to balance. This is achieved by treatment strategies that structure the disease presentation between excess and deficient parameters. Staging measures the size of the tumor and degree of spread. Stage II indicates the relative size of the neoplasm is larger in its scope, but without metastatic characteristics. This informs the clinician as to the gradation of internal blood stasis, damp-phlegm and excess heat toxin. The patient's subjective report further clarifies the diagnosis. For example, gastrointestinal cancers cause fixed, stabbing pain, a sign of blood stasis. Swelling and masses at or near the tumor site, which are visible and palpable, indicate the degree of damp-phlegm involvement. Analysis of the tongue and pulse confirm these pathologies. The tongue may be dusky-red with prickles, a damp-white coat or illustrate more *yin* deficient patterns, peeled, red tongue with fissures. The pulse may be thin, rapid, slippery or choppy. Starting from this clinical assessment, point indications that address the pathology of blood stasis with excess heat, include SP-10 (*xue hai*), LI-11 (*qu chi*) and UB-40 (*wei zhong*). With predominant damp-phlegm accumulation, classic points are effective, such as SP-9 (*yin ling quan*), Ren-9 (*shui fen*), and ST-40 (*feng long*).

The underlying deficiency of stage II-III cancers are varied in nature. As with everything in TCM, so much depends on constitution and concurrent conditions. This complexity is multifold in oncology, and patterns of deficiency are extensive. To merely address blood and *yin* deficiency at this stage is too simplistic. But it is a crucial step to the development of a more complete understanding and treatment of mid-stage cancer presentations where the disease has reached beyond its original site, threatening wider spread. This energy is abundantly *yang* in nature. This action is overacting and to balance this movement, *yin* must be nourished, and the heat must be quelled.

Treatment approaches are therefore, dual-focused: tonification and reduction. The latter strategy is executed according to the strength and specific excess pathology. The former requires a delineation of which *yin* channels are affected by the tumor itself and subsequently depleted. In patients undergoing chemotherapy we refer to the treatment structure noted above for early stage cancers in order to carefully align therapeutic techniques according to conventional side-effects and cyclical presentations. At this stage, the *yin* of the body requires nourishment. The purpose of the *Yin Wei* does precisely that; it is multifaceted in its ability to gather all of the *yin* throughout the body and return it to the Sea of *Yin*. In turn, this anchors *yang*, and in terms of neoplastic growth, perhaps it lessens the cellular activity or at least prevents an overabundance of this energy.

A significant majority of patients receive radiation therapy as a form of conventional treatment. It is used in cases when tumors are beyond surgical resection, or in combination with chemotherapy to completely eradicate disease. There are multiple ways in which radiation is delivered. External beam radiation targets solid tumors, as well as blood and lymph cancers. Brachytherapy is internal radiotherapy that places radioactive sources within the body or near the tumor to kill cancer cells. Whichever mechanism, Chinese medicine recognizes the temperature of radiation therapy as hot in nature, and this heat eradicates cancer cells and *yin*. So, while there are no cytotoxic effects caused by radiation, injury occurs on a cumulative basis to a very localized region of the body. In this case, the *Yin Wei* channel is therapeutic. This is furthered by its paired extraordinary meridian, *Yang Wei*, which reaches the superficial layers of the body treating issues of the skin. In its entirety, the *Yin Wei* engenders *yin* to nourish fluids and its pair, *Yang Wei*, extends this reach to the outer layers, where radiation burns are prominent.

The clinical guidelines for bloodletting technique emphasize its usage primarily for excess pathology not vacuity patterns. Students of Chinese medicine and seasoned practitioners have learned how to apply this method as a reducing therapy to clear heat and alleviate pain. While this is true, there is a coherent relationship between deficiency and excess patterns.

The impairment of *qi*, the presence of blood stasis, damp, phlegm or heat are all cofactors in the development of deficiency. These pathogenic evils inhibit movement, thus leading to depletion. Pricking therapy is a technique to expel the excess. In doing so, circulation is restored, and deficiency may be supplemented. This concept was taught by Dr. Henry McCann who illustrates how chronic disease, which we liken to the severity of cancer, causes Kidney essence depletion. This decline leads to an insufficiency of blood production that decreases circulation in the body and ultimately causes patterns of blood stasis.[67] Thus, pricking therapy is beneficial as a technique that simultaneously reduces and tonifies.

Acupuncture Technique: Pricking Therapy

Bloodletting, a technique within the scope of acupuncture also was also utilized in early days of Chinese medicine to rid the body of heat, toxins and disease. Accepted references to bloodletting therapy as a potent, effective modality can be found cross culturally as far back as 3,000 years ago beginning with the Egyptians all the way up to modern day India.[68] The belief in the use of bloodletting for a wide range of disorders, including deadly tumors was a part of America's medical history all the way through the 19th century that all but ended in favor of the introduction of pharmaceutical intervention.[69] Phlebotomy, as a practice of bloodletting is commonly known in Western medicine, is actually still in practice today. But it is employed with much less frequency and usually for very specific conditions such as hemochromatosis or polycythemia. However, today there are still many communities, such as in India, that adopt bloodletting as an effective treatment for anything from arthritis to cervical cancer.[70]

While the history of bloodletting typically refers to the puncturing or slicing of a vein or local swelling, TCM historically includes these methods as well as the pricking of small network vessels, such as spider nevi, and specific points on meridians like *jing-well* points. The technique of pricking

---

[67] McCann, 2014
[68] Seigworth, 1980
[69] Nickel, 2011
[70] Katz, 2014

jing-well points is what is typically taught in many American TCM schools today. The exact origins of bloodletting in TCM are unknown, however some scholars believe they may go back as far as the Oracle Bone writings from the Shang Dynasty (1600–1027).[71] Others point to the texts from the Ma Wang Dui tombs, which were sealed in 168 B.C., and its references to a *"bian,"* or lancing stone, as the possible written introduction to invasive therapies such as draining abscesses and bloodletting.[72] Without more evidence both of these thoughts remain speculation and fall secondary to the more accepted *Huang Di Nei Jing*, which was compiled between 206 B.C.E.–220 C.E., and its multiple references to bloodletting. Thus, the *Nei Jing* remains the most accepted historical text that references bloodletting in TCM.

The purpose of bloodletting therapy is twofold and may be broken down into primary and secondary functions. The first two primary functions are most well-known to practitioners: quicken the blood to transform stasis and clear heat.[73] This former approach induces movement along the vessels and channels, invigorating the blood and dispelling stasis that causes pain locally, or along the meridian. The latter opens the vessel to vent internal heat as a result of *qi, yin,* or *yang* deficiency not allowing blood to circulate properly, which creates internal pathological heat. The secondary functions are "understood as the result of a primary function or functions." They include:

1. Stops Pain
2. Resolves Toxin
3. Disperses Swellings
4. Disperses Concretions
5. Stops Itching
6. Settles and Tranquilizes
7. Opens the Orifices in Emergency Conditions
8. Resolves the Exterior[74]

---

[71] McCann, 2014
[72] Unschuld, 2003
[73] McCann, 2014
[74] ibid

Bloodletting therapy with respect to cancer treatment is dependent on the TCM diagnosis. Of the above noted functions, many are associated with the disease thus making the therapy appropriate: heat, pain, toxin, swellings, itching, and settling the spirit. Dispersing concretions is specifically indicated for cancer. A concretion is "a type of abdominal mass typically located in the lower burner and associated with pain, distension and a definite shape."[75] Other examples of specific point selections include bleeding LI-11 (*qu chi*) for esophageal cancer, or a 23-point group called *fu chao er shi san* (Bowel Nest Twenty-Three) for intestinal cancers.[76]

The technique of bloodletting is typically described as pricking the point or area on the same side of the condition being treated. We also say area because one way the bleeding method, like acupuncture, can be described as working is through a system of correspondences where the body is reflected within itself.[77] For example, it is common to bleed the veins in the area around UB-40 (*wei zhong*) for back pain or the "Liver zone" on the leg for liver issues, etc. However, in TCM there are few, if any, absolutes.

For instance, a patient we treated regularly during active cancer treatment presented with cellulitis on her foot extending onto her lower leg. This occurred nine months into recovery and is a crucial phase of rebuilding immunity and *qi*. Unfortunately, this infection presented aggressively, which impaired her ability to walk because of the pain. Her foot was easily three times its normal size. She was scheduled to see her doctor later that day but in the meantime came in for treatment. We only agreed to treat as long as she went immediately to her primary physician afterwards. Auricular method and bloodletting the *jing-wells* of the *opposite* foot was the main treatment approach. The outcome was immediately noticeable. The bleeding decreased the swollen foot to near normal size. She stood without assistance and reported very little pain while walking.

---

[75] ibid
[76] ibid
[77] McCann, 2015

This case demonstrates that pricking therapy is efficient and produces immediate and at times, dramatic results. Historically, the amount of blood varies according to theory and reflects quite a wide range. Blood is a precious substance in TCM, and therefore, some scholars teach that a few drops is therapeutic enough, versus some who would leave a bucket under the patient and walk away. The most common method in modern TCM education is to watch the color of the blood change from dark (blood stasis) to light, or bright red (heat and inflammation) to healthy red. Bloodletting requires a specific technique and should only be done by a trained practitioner. Further, the application of this therapy during cancer warrants extreme caution for deficient patients, or those taking blood thinning agents both synthetic and herbal.

Dr. McCann teaches bleeding will invigorate the Kidney and is appropriate even with deficient patterns. Careful monitoring of the pulse confirms this theory. As we have noticed, our patients' Kidney pulses strengthen when the appropriate amount of bleeding is done. Bloodletting therapy is a less common technique of acupuncture, but its long history exists not only in Chinese medicine but also throughout the world and serves to prove its relevance in a medical context.

Yang Deficiency and *Yin-Yang* Separation

The progression from *yin* deficiency syndromes in stage II-III neoplastic disease naturally unfold into combined patterns of *yang* depletion, which is one of the primary diagnoses in advanced cancer. The transition between these stages can be quite subtle. This is due to a multitude of cofactors comprised of:

- the type of cancer
- more aggressive conventional medicine regimens
- the physiological response to both.

In essence, it is a perfect storm at the cellular level within the body. Clinically, the physical, emotional and energetic effects become painfully visible. A cascade of changes, which originate from deep within the body, make their way to the surface.

Practitioners must be prepared for this transition, both in terms of clinical skill and compassionate care. This information extends from our journey as clinicians who have treated patients up until their last days. Therefore, we impart this perspective to remind practitioners in cancer care that the transformational process occurring in end stage disease goes far beyond the diagnostic assessment or technical skills. Bearing witness to the transitional phase of life to death is a remarkable experience, and as clinicians we must stay mindful and present.

The symptomatology that accompanies late-stage cancer is inherently complex. The physical side-effects and complications related to the progression of the disease dominate the overall presentation. Symptoms worsen as a result of the conventional medicine regimens, which provide a host of issues as well. Quite often there are so many interrelated side-effects, it convolutes the clinical approach. The questions we are asked most often by colleagues and interns relate to the end stage process from alleviating discomfort and improving the quality of life to prolonging it. We recognized a need for integrative content on late-stage and end-of-life care when a veteran TCM practitioner said, "I looked at my patient and just knew there was nothing I could do, so I sent her home." As a result, the material in this section is intended to rectify any doubt practitioners have in relation to therapeutic medicine in late-stage cancer.

In the private clinic, there are two distinctions among patients who present with this degree of malignancy. First, there are those previously diagnosed with cancer. As such, they may have already completed cyclical chemotherapy, and perhaps even experienced a period of remission, but the cancer had returned and metastasized. Reasons as to why recurrence occurs in some and not others are not well identified. So much is dependent on the type of cancer relative to available treatment protocols, and as always, patient constitution. In Chinese medicine, close analysis of constitutional factors provides a complete understanding of the original disease etiology, and its recurrence.

There are certain characteristics among cases of recurrence that highlight a very real concern in aspects of relapse particularly in relation to survivorship. Quite simply, once conventional treatment is completed, patients consider the acute disease eliminated and in doing so, cease various forms of complementary modalities. While we attempt to explain the integral value of self-care during the recovery phase, which follows chemotherapy or radiation regimen, a majority of patients tend to return to old behaviors and a way of life that existed prior to diagnosis. The danger in this scenario is evident by the fact that this is precisely the environment in which the disease originated. Whether improper diet, lack of exercise, overwork, stress, worry or long ignored health conditions, there is great risk returning to the scene of the crime without mindful changes to one's health.

Additionally, the impact of neoplastic disease and the treatment of it compromises the biological terrain and in essence, creates depletion; an ideal situation for an opportunistic disease to reappear. Thus, while there is great value in returning to routine, including work, family and friendships, the body is in a very delicate healing state for some time. We remind patients that one of the most significant periods of the entire cancer experience is what happens in between interventional methods, or after the cancer is no longer detected. This is when healing is directed from the defensive fight to preventative. Ironically, this is when we notice patients tend to depart from supportive therapy modalities.

By comparison, we consult with a multitude of patients who are first diagnosed at stage III-IV. Metastatic disease is present and general prognoses are poor. Cancer is treatable but not curable and survival rates depend on the type of cancer. For example, the five-year survival rate for stage IV nonsquamous cell lung cancer is less than 5%.[78] Stage IV breast cancer, however, has an estimated survival rate of 22%.[79] The complexity of the clinical approach is equal to the disease pattern in these cases. The excess pathology is well-developed, disturbing local and systemic aspects of the physical body. This excess pathogen, true to its *yang* energy, is well-motivated and unanchored by the grounding nature of *yin*. As a result, complications are extensive and cumulatively inhibit defensive mechanisms in the body.

The transition of the disease from intermediate (*yin* deficiency with heat), to late-stage (*yang* deficiency) is a visible process when it occurs. Cytotoxic therapy and radiation cause overt physical side-effects that lead to further depletion of the blood, which is a *yin* substance. A direct

---

[78] American Cancer Center, 2017
[79] ibid

consequence of deficient *yin* is untethered *yang*, which over time subtly and slowly declines because it is unchecked and burns out. An eventual separation of *yin* and *yang* results. Thus, when the malignancy surpasses the strength of the conventional methods and its host, a systemic degeneration becomes even more apparent. The complications that ensue reflect utmost disharmony, but acupuncture therapy in combination with other modalities is a valuable aspect of palliative care that treats the whole person.

The characteristics of *yang* deficiency during stage III-IV are not always classically represented. They certainly do not occur as a singular diagnostic pattern. TCM practitioners are familiar with the key features:

- lassitude
- bright-white complexion
- fatigue
- cold sensations
- pale-wet tongue
- deep, weak pulse

While these are textbooks symptoms, they are merely the underlying component to the intricate nature of late-stage cancer, which emerges in conjunction with physiological patterns that weaken the body. This decline overlaps with acute symptoms that further impair the patient's comfort. Specific conditions include cancer-related pain, gastrointestinal disturbance, abdominal and pleural ascites, dyspnea, fluctuation of fever and chills, and when a patient is moving closer towards death, delirium and compromised mental acuity. The degree to which these occur is dependent on a sequence of events that influence a systemic response in accordance with tumor pathology and location.

The following section highlights several cancer-related conditions associated with advanced disease. It is not intended to be a complete list, and while it is easy enough to indicate a symptom and recommended treatment approach, it is never quite that straightforward. The integration of TCM modalities, particularly in stage III-IV, rely upon the skill of the practitioner to see beyond the acute manifestation and observe the under-lying physical and emotional energy. It is always an interchange of excess and deficient. Therefore, for the purpose of practical application, we have included clinical strategies that have proved efficacious in collaborative medicine for our cancer patients.

Cancer-related Pain

Cancer-related pain is a common condition that plagues many patients. The location and size of the tumor has immeasurable capacity to impinge nerves and compress adjacent tissue. This creates local or regional inflammation that can become a relentless complication that affects quality of life from appetite to sleep. In Chinese medicine, *yang* deficient pain patterns are associated with concurrent *qi* deficiency in conjunction to the predominant excess pathology (blood stasis, phlegm or toxic heat). The decline of *yang* in chronic disease impairs the function of *zang-fu* organs and channels.[80] This results in lack of circulation that disrupts the blood and causes pain.

Acupuncture therapy is effective in decreasing levels of pain as part of comfort care. Emphasis on the location of the malignancy from the site of origin to its spread is the first consideration. The channels utilized in treatment can therefore correlate to the areas of stasis and pain. We refer to the previous section on resolving excess pathogenic factors associated with tumor sites. But, in order for the treatment to take effect, the *yang* must be tonified. Without supplementation, the ability of the body to drain and release the excess is reduced. Proper dredging of the channels and vessels is not motivated without the *yang*. Therefore, acupuncture points that complement this therapeutic principle are necessary.

The application of basic *yang* tonifying points create a foundation for a circulatory, pain-relieving outcome. Classic points include: Du-4 (*ming men*), Du-20 (*bai wei*), ST-36 (*zu san li*), Ren-6 (*qi hai*), KI-7 (*fu liu*), UB-23 (*shen shu*), all of which are enhanced by moxibustion therapy. The incorporation of the *Chong* meridian addresses pain in its ability to resolve excess patterns of blood stasis, as well as nourish blood. It is a meridian that functions as a conduit of circulation and tonification. As one of the eight extraordinary meridians, its efficacy is invaluable for patients in prolonged illness with moderate to severe levels of pain. For a complete discussion of the *Chong* and cancer, see the Chapter 8 on the eight extraordinary

---

[80] Peiwen, 2003

meridians. Pricking therapy of the specific channels affected by the tumor resolves excess, and as previously covered, nourishes Kidney vacuity.

Abdominal Ascites

Malignant ascites appears more frequently in intermediate and late-stage cancers of the gastrointestinal system, colon, liver, pancreas, and ovaries. It occurs with metastatic spread in the abdominal cavity that are linked to other cancers such as breast, esophageal, and leukemia. When we observe abdominal distension, which is eventually diagnosed as ascites, it is a warning sign that the body is deteriorating. The buildup of fluid in the abdominal or peritoneal cavity creates pressure on the adjacent organs causing distension and pain. In turn, patients experience nausea, vomiting and low appetite. Our patients generally state they feel quite heavy and bloated, which causes a further decline in energy. This is worsened by no desire to eat, which weakens their system and leads to cachexia.

Chinese medicine correlates this manifestation to excess damp and water accumulation in the interior. The infiltrating tumors are also comprised of blood stasis and phlegm, all of which create a trifecta of excess pathology. Underlying these patterns is the deficiency. At the *yang* depletion phase, the Spleen and Kidney are the principle organs involved. This condition is profoundly challenging to treat. The primary TCM principle focuses on tonification of the Spleen and Kidney *yang* in order to drain damp and resolve the fluid accumulation. The Western medical approach is to prescribe diuretics to promote urination and eliminate the water buildup. However, in late-stage malignancy, the fluid increases steadily and quickly. Most often patients find relief from a paracentesis. This is an outpatient procedure that extracts fluid from the abdominal cavity for immediate relief. Several liters can be drained at a time, which improves digestive and respiratory function. It is a palliative approach only as the fluid rebuilds over time. A catheter port can be placed in the abdomen to drain fluids at a more constant rate, which some patients prefer.

When this condition is present, we encourage patients to come in for acupuncture prior to a paracentesis to strengthen the *qi* and *yang* and optimize the body's response to the procedure. Symptoms that accompany *yang* deficient ascites correspond to the Spleen and Kidney. Certainly, there is abdominal distension, lack of appetite, a pale and sometimes sallow complexion, no desire to walk or move around, and difficulty laying down because of the pressure on the lungs. Patients report that they, "just can't get comfortable." Therefore, the treatment focus is to emphasize patient comfort. Acupuncture points to drain damp are effective, including: SP-9 (*yin ling quan*), LU-5 (*chi ze*), ST-40 (*feng long*), KD-10 (*yin gu*) and Ren-3 (*zhong ji*). These points can be supplemented by the *Dai* channel of the eight extraordinary meridians. The *Dai* regulates all the channels of the body, and most importantly, it is the foundation for the Spleen and Kidney meridians. Examination of the "Stomach zone" on the lower legs is warranted for pricking therapy. This region lies on the anterior ankle.[81] This technique treats symptoms associated with ascites, like abdominal pain, stomach cancers, wheezing and indigestion.[82]

Low Appetite

Low appetite that is prolonged without any period in which the patient desires food is another clinical red flag. We grow increasingly concerned during this transitional phase because malnourishment is a contributing factor in cancer death. In advanced cancer, reports indicate 60–80% of patients are cachexic and in the last 1–2 weeks of life almost 86%.[83] In early and intermediate cancers, anorexia is a cyclical symptom that occurs with chemotherapy or radiation cycles. In these regimens, appetite generally improves, and any cancer-related weight loss is amended with regular food intake. However, loss of appetite slowly evolves dangerously in prolonged illness. The cumulative effect of conventional medicine compromises the integrity of the gastrointestinal tract. Solid tumors in the gut also impair healthy digestive function.

 The decline of the Spleen and Stomach over the course of the disease is the center point for *yang* vacuity patterns related to appetite and digestion. It is important to distinguish the degree of anorexia according to stage of illness. In stage I-II, low appetite correlates to Spleen and Stomach

---

[81] McCann, 2014

[82] ibid

[83] Cancer Cachexia Hub, 2018

deficiency due to conventional methods that inhibit the normal function of transforming food and fluids to produce blood and *qi*. Secondary to this pattern is nausea and anxiety causing low appetite, which more closely identifies with Liver *qi* overacting on the middle *jiao*. The mechanism of anorexia in advanced cancer correlates to Spleen *qi* deficiency and Kidney *yang* depletion. This distinction is necessary when devising treatment principles according to the clinical stage of the illness.

In advanced stage with dysregulated digestion, the treatment strategy is to warm and nourish Kidney *yang* and tonify Spleen *qi*. This is an approach that alleviates patient discomfort, encourages energy production and stabilizes the physiological response to the disease progression. In combination with moxibustion, the following points are recommended: ST-36 (*zu san li*), UB-20 (*pi shu*), UB-21 (*wei shu*), Du-4 (*ming men*), UB-23 (*shen shu*), Ren-12 (*zhong wan*), LV-13 (*zhang men*). To the seasoned TCM practitioner, these are relatively obvious point combinations. We reiterate these principles and strategies to illustrate the importance of measuring the patient's physical phase with the disease stage. There are myriad avenues in treatment strategies, but above all, it is clinical discernment that facilitates the appropriate method of patient-centered care. And in end-stage illness, palliative methodology is the foremost endeavor of any practitioner in cancer management.

End of Life: The Separation of *Yin* and *Yang*

It is an immeasurable privilege to provide Chinese medicine for patients who have endured the journey of cancer. In an ideal world, all of these individuals win the fight. We have hope that someday this is the reality, but until then we continue to work within our scope and care for our patients who are dying. The final stages of death are accompanied by incredible strength and grace. In Chinese medicine, we are taught to observe the eyes, which house the spirit, or *Shen*. There is a soft, subtle transition that takes place when a patient is in transition from life to death. When the clinician establishes rapport with patients and their caregivers, an energetic bond develops creating a palpable connection of compassion and care. This is the most difficult aspect of cancer management. When patients with whom we have encouraged and treated for short or long periods of time, succumb to the illness.

To bear witness to the dying process challenges even the most grounded provider. Tai Lahans, a modern scholar of Chinese medical oncology states it aptly, "The living and dying experience becomes a relationship between the patient and provider; this relationship begins early in the medical relationship and is defined often by very early connections and understanding that evolve as part of the trust for and openness to each other."[84] The clinical treatments that precede the final stages of death are refined and simple. If the patient is still mobile and is accompanied to the clinic, there is an opportunity to address physical discomforts to lessen pain or improve breathing, but frequently patients begin to talk about death. Regardless of faith or spirituality, patients become quite present to this reality and begin to reflect on life and their passing. This energy is often encompassed by acceptance. Of course, dying from cancer is not desired, but for some, after an arduous fight, there is a readiness to let go. This aligns with the Kidney deficiency at play, the emotional energy associated with this *fu* organ, the *zhi* (will) is declining.

In this dynamic, the therapeutic options are limited. The *qi* and blood of the body are weak, *yin* and *yang* are deficient. Measuring the presence and quality of the Spleen and Stomach pulse indicate the degree of vitality that remains. In advanced disease, the resilience of this pulse position is indeed an indicator of progression. We closely track the quality of this pulse throughout treatment but more closely at the end of life. When the middle pulse has lost its strength and can no longer be felt, the patient is close to death. Thus, it is not the role of the practitioner to strongly tonify and deter the progression. Herein is the opportunity to provide energetic palliative care. Perhaps it is in death and dying that the art of Chinese medicine reflects it truest energy, and within this, we depend on the eight extraordinary meridians. Each channel corresponds to a physical and emotional bond within the self. Because the meridians run at deeper levels of the body, they are more closely linked to the essence and emotional terrain of the person, present and past.

---

[84] Lahans, 2003

The separation of *yin* and *yang* is death, which occurs as part of life's continuum where the emotional spirit has resided throughout. The transformative process of dying can be nurtured through the *Dai, Chong or Yang Wei* channels, all of which are inherently connected to the physiological body. Each is a conduit in balancing emotional energy relative to the physical. The *Chong* is where the true self resides through its connection to the Kidneys and Heart. For patients who are introspective in the final stages, a *Chong* treatment supports this period of self-reflection. The *Yang Wei* is the meridian of encouragement. Its energy helps to move forward and not remain stuck and resistant but accept the path ahead. Of these, however, the *Dai* is our clinical gem. This channel connects to all meridians, it relates to the Spleen and Kidney *qi*. It nourishes the Spleen to calm overthinking and worry, which happens as a byproduct when the Spleen is weak. Similarly, when the Kidney *qi* is weak, fear is present, which is an emotion quite central to the process of dying. The psychological components of the *Dai* connect to feelings of resentment, inability to let go of the past, trying to control life and not allowing it to unfold. When the patient is ready for death, the energy of the *Dai* channel meets the needs of the spirit to gracefully pass.

We have observed profound responses in home-care visits, often at the request of caregivers, by treating the patient with acupuncture on two or three points to nourish *yin* and calm the spirit. The uprising of the *yang*, often understood as the last push of this energy before it separates from *yin*, can also be anchored. This helps to reduce delirium and anxiety. SP-6 (*san yin jiao*) and KI-3 (*tai xi*) nourish blood and root the *yin*. The technique is slight: mild tonification with shallow insertion. Gentle moxibustion pairs well with these points to supplement, warm and nourish.

The relationship that develops among patients and providers is an integral component in the cancer journey. It is important to recognize the value of integrating Chinese medicine modalities to alleviate the physical complications, but true to the nature of the practice, it is compassionate care that drives the medicine. Its innate connection to the emotional and spiritual body comes full circle at the end of life. This extends from the TCM doctor toward the patient, their family, friends and caregivers. We recall the passing of a special individual who we treated for almost a year for stage IV pancreatic cancer, whose wife accompanied him at each appointment.

When he transitioned to hospice and in the last few days, she asked if we would provide one last treatment for him at home. He passed away hours before we arrived, and when she called to inform our office, we asked how we could support her, and she said, "Please come over, we need ritual." On the floor of her living room, we treated five family members who were all sprawled out, sharing stories, laughing and crying.

That is the heart of Chinese medicine.

References

American Cancer Society. (2017). *Breast Cancer Survival Rates*. Retrieved September 25, 2018, from https://www.cancer.org/cancer/breast-cancer/understanding-a-breast-cancer-diagnosis/breast-cancer-survival-rates.html

American Cancer Society. (2017). Non-Small Cell Lung Cancer Survival Rates, by Stage. Retrieved August 14, 2018, from https://www.cancer.org/cancer/non-small-cell-lung-cancer/detection-diagnosis-staging/survival-rates.html

Cancer Cachexia Hub. (n.d.). Epidemiology, Cancer Cachexia. Retrieved October 17, 2018, from http://www.cancercachexia.com/epidemiology-hcp

Katz, K. (2014). *Leeches are Sucking Their Way Back Into Modern Medicine*. Retrieved January 3, 2015, from Rasmussen College: http://www.rasmussen.edu/degrees/health-sciences/blog/leeches-in-modern-medicine/

Lahans, T. (2007). *Integrating Conventional and Chinese Medicine in Cancer Care: A Clinical Guide*. Philadelphia, PA: Churchill Livingstone Elsevier.

McCann, H. (2014). *Pricking the Vessels: Bloodletting Therapy in Chinese Medicine*. Philadelphia: Singing Dragon.

Maciocia, G. (2005). *The foundations of Chinese medicine: A comprehensive text for acupuncturists and herbalists* (2nd ed.). Edinburgh: Elsevier Churchill Livingstone.

Nickel, J. C. (2011). Bloodletting and the Management of Localized Prostate Cancer. *Canadian Urological Association Journal* , 159–160.

Peiwen, L. (2003). *Management of Cancer with Chinese Medicine*. St. Albans, Herts, UK: Donica Publishing Ltd.

Seigworth, G. R. (1980). *A Brief History of Bloodletting*. Retrieved January 3, 2015, from PBS: http://www.pbs.org/wnet/redgold/basics/bloodlettinghistory.html

Unschuld, P. U. (trans) (2003). *Huang Di Nei Jing Su Wen*. Berkeley: University of California Press.

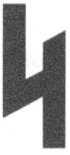

Moxibustion Therapy

"When I feel the heat, I see the light."
Everett Dirksen

Similar to the other modalities that comprise Chinese medicine, there is not an exact, universally accepted date of when the technique of moxibustion originated, or when it was integrated into the theory of TCM. The knowledge and skillful application of this modality could render its very own book. It is an honored modality in countries like Japan, where doctors of moxibustion rely entirely on this heat therapy in their practice. We can only hope practitioners of the West regard it someday with as much reverence as our colleagues do abroad. For the purpose of this book, we begin with an overview of its historical background, and then define the characteristics and purpose of moxibustion as it relates to cancer management in clinical settings. The final section will present clinical experience relevant to common conditions observed with cancer patients and the benefit of moxibustion as a singular modality for their case.

A Brief History of Moxibustion

Varied stories of folklore associate the origins of moxibustion with the Brahmins of India as far back as the 8th century B.C., while some guess its origins are loosely associated with the discovery of fire.[85] To date, depending on one's interpretation of translations, the oldest known writing that references

---

[85] Merlin, 2012

moxa therapy comes from either the Warring States period (475–221 B.C.) by two separate philosophers, Mengzi and Zhuangzi, or from the *Zuo zhuan*, compiled roughly from 770 B.C.–476 B.C., during the Spring and Autumn period. The first discourse on moxa that appears within the paradigm of medicine is found in the Mawangdui text, likely written between 300 and 200 B.C. There is not a single point of origin that has been identified, but in Chapter 12 of the classical text *Huang Di Nei Jing Su Wen*, it states moxibustion as definitely "…originating in the North," which corresponds to the cold climate of the region.[86] These facts reveal the strong likelihood that moxibustion predates acupuncture though it is far less recognized as a valuable form of therapy. The term "moxa," which we use regularly in modern day is essentially an abbreviation of moxibustion. It was actually coined in a report referencing a direct moxibustion technique published in Amsterdam in 1674.[87] Interestingly, it comes from a Dutch clergyman who experienced relief after the burning of a "wool-like" substance on his knee for the treatment of gout.[88] Historical references indicate the use of moxa was an integral tool for physicians. In the canon of acupuncture, known as the *Lingshu*, Chapter 73 states in cases when needling does not yield results, moxibustion can be effective and should be used.[89]

What is Moxibustion?

Moxibustion is a technique that utilizes the herb mugwort. In TCM, this herb is called *ai ye* (either Artemisia Vulgaris or Artemisiae Argyi is typically used) and functions as an external therapy to warm, clear heat, or fumigate/steam specific areas of the body. Although *ai ye* is the most common herb used in moxibustion, sometimes other substances are combined with the goal of creating a smokeless material, such as the case with charcoal. Or, other medicinal ingredients are included like *deng xin cao* (junci medulla) to enhance therapeutic applications for example. But it is mugwort in its most pure form that elicits potent heat with effective results. This also

---

[86] Unschuld, 2002

[87] Merlin, 2012

[88] ibid

[89] Wang, 2007

eliminates concerns of other chemical byproducts that burn along with the mugwort. Moxa is performed on meridians or acupoints on the body to influence a change in symptom presentation, for both acute and chronic conditions. Over the two thousand years that it has been in existence, its clinical applications have become extremely refined, indicating its vast range of therapeutic abilities. First, we will explore the purpose of moxibustion therapy, and then focus on three primary techniques frequently categorized as direct, indirect and semi-direct forms of therapy.

Therapeutic Function and Purpose of Moxibustion

Classical functions of moxibustion are extensive. Its therapeutic purpose aims to warm the channels, tonify *qi* and *yang*, expel cold and damp, move *qi* and blood. Its warming and nourishing properties positively influence the body's response to stress whether emotional or physical injury, thereby preventing disease or limiting disease progression. This can translate to anything from orthopedic concerns including numbness, swelling and pain, to digestive ailments like diarrhea. Probably the most significant function, one that is recognized and valued by the profession at large is its known ability to optimize the immune system. In TCM oncology, it is this purpose and function of moxibustion that deems it inherently valuable and an integral component to treatment.

To further this understanding toward evidence-based medicine, there are several informal studies from Asia that have provided some insight on this immuno-enhancing effect. By and large, the Japanese have led the way in the consistent modern analysis of moxibustion dating back to the famous study in 1929 by Dr. Shimetaro Hara on the effects of moxibustion on ST-36 (*zu san li*) to raise white blood cell count. A different study by Dr. Yoshiaki Ohmura reported that moxa at ST-36 (*zu san li*) may positively affect the lymph nodes and the release of natural killer cells, which in turn could mean good news in the treatment of cancer. A 2004 study out of Korea seems to corroborate the increase in natural killer cell cytotoxicity from direct moxa also on this acupoint.[90] The degree of acceptance of these and other studies is debatable even by Chinese medicine standards, but at the

---

[90] Merlin, 2012

very least, they beg for more focused research in the area of moxibustion. It also provides reasoning for a greater attempt by modern practitioners to employ specific protocols to address the frequent side-effects of conventional cancer treatment like fatigue, neutropenia and low appetite.

The action of moxibustion as a heat therapy is *yang* in nature. By extension, *qi* is *yang* in nature, and therefore it is reasonable that moxibustion can increase the production of *qi* as well. It is a known principle in TCM that *yin* can transform into *yang* and vice versa. Thus, depending on the technique applied, the properties of moxa warm and tonify the *qi* and/or *yang* of the body. Moxibustion is said to have originated in Northern China, a region that tends toward cold temperatures where moxa would be an invaluable therapy. Thus, in classical texts, many early references to moxibustion therapy identify the use of this heat therapy for *yin* syndromes. Interestingly, Chinese medicine principles observe that the early stages of cancer align mostly with cold patterns, and late-stage with *qi* and *yang* deficiency with concurrent pathogenic heat accumulations. In both stages, moxibustion is warranted. By contrast to its strengthening function, mugwort can also reduce heat and clear inflammation. This is an approach, which is similar to "like treats like"; this will be illustrated in further detail later in this chapter. Clinical understanding of this potent heat therapy has evolved over the last couple of millennia, and as a result, its efficacy has grown to include an ever larger number of syndromes including cold, hot, internal or external (physical) levels.

Information regarding the quantity and dosing of moxibustion therapy is less available in classical texts and modern studies. As dedicated moxa practitioners, we find this very frustrating. While we respect our colleagues in Asia who have at least attempted some form of a scientific study on moxa's medicinal value, the reports are vague on dosage and poorly designed. For example, one may read classical Chinese texts that recommend 300 cones of moxa of a non-specific size over an unknown number of treatments for a mostly vague condition to find success. While hundreds of cones on a point or area may be of value and provide dramatic clinical results, the time, intensity, and possible disfigurement of such a treatment often makes it impractical in modern clinical practice. Japanese methods, on the contrary, advocate the cumulative effects of moxibustion and cite the importance of daily treatment with few cones being best.

This last approach aligns with the inherent concept of prevention in TCM, and one that is adaptable as a lifestyle. Meaning that the small daily changes that a person makes has a greater long-term synergistic effect on one's health and wellness over the occasional stronger treatments. Of course, this approach presents its own difficulties. Our very busy Western society is already challenged by scheduling patients frequently enough to garner the value of cumulative treatments with needles much less moxa. Ultimately the onus is on the practitioners to employ methods and techniques of moxibustion that they are comfortable with.

Direct Moxibustion

The direct form of moxa can be utilized for tonification or sedation. For Western Chinese medicine practitioners, this technique is less frequently utilized due to the potential risk of scarring. Ironically, classical literature references "scarring moxa." This was performed for the purpose of producing a "moxa flower," essentially a scar. The conceptual foundation of this technique was that the "flower" would trap the heat thereby continuing to stimulate the point until the flower healed, thus prolonging the treatment effect. As a result of this possible outcome, direct moxa is not permitted under scope of practice in some states, and practitioners are therefore less likely to risk upsetting patients, or even worse, contend with a malpractice suit. Chinese medicine schools touch on this method very briefly. Therefore, practitioners do not become skilled or comfortable using it in practice. We have found that by clearly explaining the method, how it is being used and for what purpose, patients are accepting and find it quite soothing.

The moxa product used in the direct technique varies according to its therapeutic goal. Tonification merits the use of aged, refined moxa (golden in color and soft in texture), while reducing techniques utilize green, coarse moxa wool to generate higher heat levels. In tonification techniques, the moxa wool is formed into loose, supple cones. This softness lessens the heat intensity and causes the mugwort to burn at a faster rate as not to build up too much heat on the point. The size of the pieces varies and can be as small as a thread or a grain of rice, and slightly larger and similar to the size of a Hershey's Kiss. Burn cream or moxa balm can be applied as a barrier between the skin and moxa, which also provides a mild adhesive the cone can stick to on the skin. Once placed on the acupoint, the moxa cone is carefully lit with an incense stick to allow for a slow and controlled burn. It may burn entirely down to meet the skin or extinguished by the practitioner once the patient reports a warming sensation. A rice grain-sized cone is extinguished with quick placement of the practitioner's finger on the cone, or with larger style cones, forceps are used to lift the cone off the skin and immediately place in a cup of water. This method is repeated in odd numbers (1, 3, 5, 7, etc.) according to the classical concept of tonification.

By contrast, if reducing methods are indicated for cases of excess pathology, such as damp accumulation, or *qi* and blood stagnation, the direct method requires tightly packed cones formed by coarse, less refined moxa. In alignment with this principle, the cones are therefore larger in size allowing the wool to generate higher heat levels with greater capacity to clear stagnation and draw out internal heat. During application, the practitioner may gently blow on the lit cones to produce more heat at a faster burn rate. To determine dosage, the practitioner palpates for a change in texture and tone of the tissue or area being treated to assess for the anticipated change. An example of this is demonstrated in the treatment of radiation fibrosis syndrome later in this chapter.

Indirect Moxibustion

Indirect moxa techniques are the most common in modern day practice. This is likely due to the fact that the indirect form is the predominant method taught in Chinese medicine programs. It is also recognized as an easier, efficient tool of moxa application with reduced risk of burns. "Smokey" or smokeless sticks are identified in each of our clinic treatment rooms, the moxa scent permeates the atmosphere, which our patients have likened to healing and rest. Before we explore the clinical techniques for practitioners, it is important to mention a valuable component to indirect moxa. This technique, perhaps the only mode of TCM modalities and tools can be taught to patients as daily self-care. It is simple enough to explain the reasons behind this heat therapy, provide a complimentary moxa stick, demonstrate the techniques, and give an illustration of point locations and protocols. We like to say it is comparable to free dental floss at a teeth cleaning; it is easy, therapeutic and most importantly, preventative medicine.

This can have a powerful effect on empowering the patient to take part in a small aspect of their health and healing. After many years of encouraging patients to perform moxibustion at home, those who do, share that it is a comfortable, nurturing ritual they rely upon and notice a positive shift not only in physical energy levels, but serves to calm and center them as well thereby supporting the emotional energetic root.

The indirect moxibustion method is less technical and easily learned through practice. For the tonification method, the trick is to apply an even, consistent heat over the acupoint. Because of variations in anatomy and internal health, the quantity of time varies. For example, ST-36 (*zu san li*) typically requires an average of 10 minutes of steady, mild heat stimulation to yield a potent, nourishing effect. Too often we observe practitioners wave the moxa stick over a point for a minute or two as if is a magic wand. And while sometimes we joke to patients that it is, for the purpose of therapeutic benefits, technique and timing are crucial. Five minutes is typically the minimum amount of time and 15 minutes as a maximum. In addition to the magic wand approach, we observe interns or new practitioners in a hurry who rush the treatment. They place the stick too close to the skin and rapidly heat the point, which then becomes a reducing technique in total opposition to tonification goals. Another undesirable outcome of overheating the point is the introduction of excess heat into the channel.

The heat intensity should be monitored by the placement of two fingers on either side of the point. Explaining to patients who may be nervous about heat exposure that "we'll feel the intensity of the heat before you will" can alleviate concerns. This is particularly crucial in cases of neuropathy with predominant numbness, or patients with dysregulated temperature and internal cold. In either instance, the patient may not recognize the strength of the heat on their skin, which can lead to unnecessary burning. To modulate the quality of therapeutic heat, the moxa stick is pulled away from the point, followed by placing the fingers of the supporting hand on the point with gentle pressure. This helps to trap the heat as well as dull the intensity for patient comfort. If the surface of the skin is becoming uncomfortably warm for the patient, but the therapeutic effects have not been reached, then the stick should be lifted further away to lessen the intensity of the heat but continue a mild stimulation. Timing and dosage is determined by palpation and can be discerned by assessing a change of skin tone signaling end of treatment. In addition to palpation, observing a pinkish quality to the skin around the acupoint indicates proper amount of heat has been applied.

The smokey forms of moxa are a contentious issue among those in the profession who use this modality regularly. These sticks create smoke as a byproduct, which has led some practitioners toward smokeless moxa poles (charcoal based), compromising the potency of the heat for a more treatment-friendly environment. Smokey moxa is derived mainly from pure mugwort, full of volatile oils and therapeutic properties that are as medicinal in nature as the degree of heat it produces. There are no additives or other ingredients in these pure moxa polls, therefore they burn much like an herb or plant would, but with an exponentially higher degree of heat, which is precisely the medicinal component practitioners are seeking to extract in treatment. The utilization of a charcoal-based moxa stick, in order to limit smoke exposure, lessens the effectiveness of this modality. This is illustrated by a study comparing the intensity of radiation (mV) between several moxa materials. The results indicated the traditional moxa pole burned at a rate of 43,300 mV compared to its counterpart, the charcoal-infused smokeless moxa stick that burned at a rate of 31 mV.[91] Given this research, we lend ourselves toward smokey moxa to garner the most potent therapeutic outcome.

There are numerous studies on the efficacy of acupuncture, and perhaps even more so within integrative oncology program development. By contrast, moxibustion is hardly known or discussed, rarely implemented, and therefore, never researched. However, we identified a small study exploring the effects of smoke from moxibustion. A study that assessed the potential risk of inhaling extensive amounts of moxa was performed by Wheeler and Coppock, who found "...no immediate concerns from moxibustion use therapeutically."[92] To further this report, the smoke in moxibustion is thought to have antibacterial properties as well. Historically, it was burned in some Chinese hospitals as a way to clean the air.

Other than the moxa sticks, indirect forms of heat therapy are also attained by warm needle technique. In this method, a small ball of moxa is attached to the needle handle and burned in order to penetrate the heat

[91] Merlin, 2012
[92] Wheeler, 2009

into the needle, and eventually into the acupoint. Similar to direct moxa, this does carry the risk of burns, as the positioning of the moxa must be stable and watched carefully. Given the heightened sensitivity of cancer patients, as well as the likelihood that the skin has been compromised due to surgery or chemotherapy side effects, warm needle technique is rarely used in clinic and highly cautioned.

By comparison, the "moxa box" is a method that is a staple in our practice, particularly for cancer patients, due to its deep, penetrating heat that strongly nourishes the *qi* and *yang*. When cancer patients express needle sensitivity, or we determine their pulses are too weak to even receive acupuncture, we use the moxa box. It is essentially a three-by-five-by-six-inch box. There is a mesh net that rests in the box where the moxa is placed. Medium-grade moxa is sufficient and is gently rolled and placed inside the box where it is lit on one end and covered with a lid that is open just enough for smoke to seep out and for air to circulate. The rate of burn and intensity of the moxibustion can be regulated by adjusting the opening of the lid. This approach is a gentle form of moxa that can be done for an extended period of time, approximately 20–40 minutes.

The most common placement of the moxa box is below the navel and centered on *Ren-6* (*qi hai*). This is a profoundly nourishing treatment, and one that allows the patient to rest but can also control the heat intensity by picking up the box and placing it above the navel when the heat is too intense. The smoke produced is pungent, and moxa heavy treatments require an open window or air ventilation of some kind. When applied appropriately, the moxa box will cause a definitive increase in energy. It is important that patients understand that despite this immediate surge, continuing to rest is paramount in order to conserve the energy and let it take root. Without this warning, patients will harness that moxa power and attempt to do things they haven't been able to, and this will eliminate the therapeutic results. Thus, the challenge of the moxa box therapy is to allow its benefits to unfold systematically throughout the day and rebuild the *qi*. Otherwise the beneficial effects are voided, and it is akin to attempting to fill a cup with a hole in it.

Semi-direct moxibustion

Semi-direct moxibustion is also referred to as "isolating substance moxibustion," which falls under the indirect form of moxibustion category. This method, as the name implies, uses a substance between the skin and the mugwort. All manner of substances have been used to perform this method of moxibustion. The most common include the more popular herbs from the TCM pharmacopeia such as fresh ginger and salt. Typically, an isolating substance is used to either moderate the heat at the point or to impart some of the medicinal properties of the herb into the point to enhance treatment. For example, a slice of fresh ginger with moxa over *Ren*-8 (*shen que*) warms *yang* and treats deficient cold syndromes in the middle *jiao* by virtue of the ginger being a warm, cold-expelling herb. By comparison, mugwort placed upon salt on *Ren*-8 (*shen que*) alleviates diarrhea or pain due to Kidney deficiency. Salt is related to the Kidneys in TCM, which serves to modulate the function of the heat therapy and direct it toward the Kidney energy. As a conduit, salt penetrates heat quickly and so effectively that it can cause discomfort or shift an intended tonifying treatment into reducing.

In addition to the more common herbal ingredients such as ginger and salt, "cakes" are also made from powdered herbs and used to isolate moxa. For an herbalist interested in compounding plant materials, this is a superb method to facilitate specific semi-direct moxa techniques. The thickness of the substance or herb can vary widely depending on the technique being performed but is usually anywhere from a couple millimeters to a quarter of an inch thick. If using fresh ginger, as in the example above, it is best to poke several small holes in it to allow the heat to easily pass through.

Dosage in semi-direct approaches depends on the desired therapeutic outcome. As is the case with all methods, classical teachings indicate tonification is facilitated by an odd number of moxa cones, and an even number for reducing. While we respect these teachings, the reality is that not every practitioner follows these traditions. Clinical experience is influenced by a variety of factors. So while those classical approaches are valuable, we align techniques with the pulse, palpation and observation of the skin tone and color to discern therapeutic dosages.

Moxibustion for *Yin* Deficiency

Palpation is an essential skill because it illustrates the diagnostic quality of an acupoint in order to determine proper moxa technique. The dominant hand gently presses the point to assess for taut skin or a mild depression.

With *yin* deficient patterns, the skin may be slightly raised or actually convexed, think of deficient heat rising or steaming the skin upward. As a more complex palpatory diagnostic, it is possible to identify "the point within the point" at a relatively deeper level similar to a grain of sand.

With direct moxibustion, rice grain-sized cones are especially effective because of its focused and penetrating heat. However, larger sized cones will also strongly tonify and are generally easier to work with. For *yin* deficient points, a rice grain-sized moxa cone is placed directly upon it and lit. As the moxa burns, the practitioner aligns their pointer finger and thumb around the cone in preparation to press the skin on either side of the cone with relatively firm pressure. This is done because *yin* deficient points reside at a deeper level, and this technique invites the point toward the surface and receive the heat therapy to nourish *yin*. After the moxa is extinguished, firm pressure is applied over the point to trap the heat and avoid dispersion.

Moxibustion for *Yang* Deficiency

The skill of palpation also applies for *yang* deficient points, but there is certainly a significant difference to the quality of the point compared to *yin* deficient points. *Yang* vacuity points feel flaccid and soft. The temperature of the skin also may feel relatively cooler. While tracing a meridian to confirm point location, the guiding finger will "fall into a vacant hole" compared to the gritty sensation in *yin* deficient points. However, in this deeper concave presentation, the point is actually at a shallower level because *yang* characteristics are inherently superficial to *yin*. This palpation requires a softer touch much like a sweeping movement of the fingers that may catch upon the point. In *yang* deficient acupoints, it is possible to identify the precise aspect of the deficiency through careful palpation.

Therapeutic treatment of *yang* deficient points requires a "tenting" method with rice grain-sized cones. This technique reduces the oxygen to slow the burn. This is important for two reasons:

- It lessens the heat intensity.
- It fills the *yang* deficient point with potent heat to tonify *yang*.

Tenting utilizes two fingers on the dominant hand. They press together firmly and hover over the moxa as it burns. Careful observation indicates a slower burn rate compared to *yin* deficient pressing technique. Other than tenting over the point, the practitioner can also press gently on either side of the cone straight down. Do not pinch under the cone. We have practiced a myriad of techniques with different moxa products, sizes and shapes. This method has proven effective in the clinical experience time and again because rice grain-sized cones focus the heat and are deeply penetrating. The larger cones are less directed, thereby affecting more of the *yang* and *qi* level at the surface of the point. For the purpose of introducing practitioners to these methods, we encourage beginning with larger cones and exploring the shape, sizes and technique before working with smaller mugwort cones.

To summarize, the above techniques are differentiated by *yin* and *yang* characteristics. In *yin*, points are deeper, and the goal is to bring the heat up to meet the point and maximize the outcome. In *yang* acupoints are more superficial, and the technique uses a milder burn at a slower rate to allow the *qi* to build. This methodology is intended to maximize the therapeutic effect in a shorter amount of time though not mandatory and can be achieved with indirect moxa applications as well.

Moxibustion for Excess Patterns

In addition to the primary *yin/yang* deficiencies that occur in cancer presentations, there is also excess pathology. In TCM oncology, these pathogenic factors include *qi* stagnation, blood stasis, damp or phlegm and toxic heat. Palpable tumors, edema, masses or swelling with redness indicate excess conditions that have accumulated often as a result of depletion. It is imperative that the skilled clinician follows diagnostic measures to reach an appropriate Chinese medicine diagnosis and treatment principle before applying moxibustion to excess patterns or conditions.

Excess conditions are easily identifiable within points or on areas of the body. With a moderate degree of pressure, palpation will reveal a firm or soft damp accumulation with relative size, such as a small mass. The temperature of the skin can indicate degrees of excess heat patterns and suggest the duration of chronic, long-term stagnation, but in opposition to heat, the skin may feel cool and indicate cold-damp syndromes. Typically, excess patterns are easy to distinguish with careful palpation and offer visible characteristics, such as edema beneath the point.

Moxibustion for excess conditions does not require the technique nuances that deficient points demand. Stagnation of *qi* and blood, or accumulation of damp and phlegm focus the treatment approach on promoting circulation. This enables the dispersion of the pathogen (heat or damp) and/or invigorating (*qi* and blood). Thus, a reducing moxa technique creates high levels of cumulative heat, whether through applications of cones or with an indirect moxa stick. The goal is to break up or expel the excess and not allow it to be retained. Therefore the treated point or area does not need to be covered after the heat therapy.

Moxibustion Applications for Cancer Management: Neutropenia, Fatigue, Radiation Fibrosis

In cancer management, we address symptoms related to the disease at many different stages with varying degrees of presentations. Moxibustion is arguably one of the most flexible, useful and dynamic modalities with an ability to soothe, nourish and provide relief to an individual enduring the harsh effects of the disease and conventional treatments. Its powerful ability to tonify provides endless opportunity to harness the patient's innate ability to heal and encourage a stronger fight. As mentioned, the function of moxibustion works best when applied in small, frequent dosages or treatments. We often explain to patients that Chinese medicine's capacity to work is similar to the activity of running and jumping. Consider this, if you were to jump over a hurdle, are you likely to stand and jump or get a running start? In order to launch yourself over the hurdle with grace and agility, you get a running start. That is to say, many small steps are inherent to a leap forward. TCM in general, and specifically moxa, is similar. In our clinic, each cancer patient receives moxa therapy during their session. We also frequently hear, "Oh good, time for moxa," which speaks to how well it is received and while the mechanism is not always as understandable to the patient, they are drawn to its healing. TCM practitioners must encourage these tiny steps of healing through small, effective doses of this potent, therapeutic herb.

The section that follows demonstrates the versatility of mugwort based on clinical techniques that we have identified as most effective and relatively easy to incorporate with no adverse consequences. Note that this section does not provide a complete list and commentary on the varied physical presentations that accompany cancer. This book would be endless if that were the case. Instead, the material focuses on three Western conditions that often stem from conventional cancer treatment. In order to provide a baseline of integrative content for readers with a Western or Eastern medical background, each condition is defined through its own medical lens. This leads toward relevant TCM diagnosis, methods of moxibustion and recommended techniques. Our intention is to inform the reader on the merits of moxa therapy, as well as to inspire the TCM practitioner to think outside the box and to become more comfortable and adept in utilizing for complex diseases, such as cancer.

Neutropenia

Neutropenia is a condition that will likely occur for patients undergoing radiation or chemotherapy regimens. Within the bone marrow, three types of cells are produced: red blood cells (RBC), white blood cells (WBC), and platelets. The term myelosuppression indicates a decrease in any one or in all of these cells, which are highly sensitive to irradiation and cytotoxic drugs. Of these, neutrophils are a type of WBC responsible for fighting infection. The cumulative effect of cytotoxic therapies can cause a decline of WBC. Thresholds can vary, but typically when counts measure less than 1,500 neutrophils per microliter of blood, oncologists postpone treatment until the level rises to 3,000. This can become a very dangerous condition that requires close monitoring and attention.

It is important to reiterate that a primary goal of Chinese medical oncology is to support the patient with the intention of maintaining conventional medicine treatment plans. Postponement of chemotherapy not only prolongs the rather aggressive course of care for the patient, causing stress and frustration, but it also provides opportunity for cellular proliferation. This calls for the restorative capacity of moxibustion. Treatments can be particularly useful when risk of infection is cautioned, and oncologists or patients are concerned about needle treatments. Although lab value analysis is not central to the Oriental medicine practice, it is advantageous to review lab values for chronic or persistent myelosuppressive conditions. While we cannot scientifically measure values of *qi* or blood, it is possible, and we argue necessary, for the TCM provider to review labs to stay informed of hematopoietic function of the bone marrow. This data can be a useful guide to refine treatment approaches, which leads to better outcomes and illustrates the essence of TCM integrative oncology.

Chinese Medicine Patterns

Chinese medicine has the ability to interpret modern biomedical conditions and align them with the classical concepts from which the medicine is derived. The condition of neutropenia is no different. In both concepts of medicine, blood is a vital physiological substance integral to good health. In myelosuppression, the body is essentially overtaxed compromising the production of blood cells in the bone marrow. This taxation is central to the TCM pattern that corresponds to neutropenia, referred to as blood deficiency (*xue xu*). It is important to note that blood deficiency in Chinese medicine does not equate to the biological aspect of anemia. The TCM understanding of blood formation is rooted in Chinese medicine theory and a fundamental component to treating blood-related patterns.

Chinese medicine reveres the Kidney organ. It holds *essence*, governs the bones and is responsible for marrow production, and through this pattern, there is some crossover between the Eastern and Western concepts of blood. However, in TCM most of the emphasis is put on the Spleen as the main producer of blood and secondarily, the Kidney. The Spleen is one of the main organs of digestion, where nutrition is converted to blood and other vital substances in the body according to Chinese medicine theory. When this becomes weakened, whether through diet, stress or disease, the Spleen becomes deficient itself, and the healthy production of blood is impaired. This is evident through side effects associated with conventional cancer treatment. Symptoms of myelosuppression and blood deficiency include fatigue, generalized weakness, low appetite, a feeling of cold and susceptibility to infection.

This diagnosis can manifest differently in clinic according to stage of disease and individual constitution. A young individual experiencing an early diagnosis and first occurrence may have labs that indicate neutropenia but report feeling only mild low energy but continue to eat and sleep relatively well. Often these patients, in lieu of postponing, are more apt to advocate for continuing chemotherapy in an effort to complete the cycles as quickly as possible. By comparison, the older individual or a person with metastatic spread who has endured numerous rounds of cytotoxic therapy will physically present with symptoms of lethargy, dizziness, body aches and inability to fight off a cold. The clinical skill to observe the degree of neutropenia or blood deficiency without labs is crucial. In order to strengthen this weakness, the treatment principle is to nourish blood. This concept of nourishing equates to an aspect of healing the body. This is not too dissimilar to the Western concept of blood in which white blood cells fight to heal infection, and red blood cells help heal soft tissue.

Moxibustion for Neutropenia

The versatility of moxibustion allows for its application on different areas of the body, corresponding to influential regions or specific acupuncture points. Of the myriad of options, and for the purpose of concise and accessible information, this section will focus on basic techniques proven to be effective for neutropenia or other forms of myelosuppression. The most familiar acupuncture point, one used extensively in vacuity patterns, and classified by a physician from the Jin dynasty, Ma Dan-yang, as one of the most vital acupuncture points is Stomach 36 (*zu san li*).[93] By virtue of its numerous classical indications, this acupoint has been relied upon extensively and rightfully so, particularly for its function of increasing *qi* and our modern understanding of immunity. This occurs by way of its actions to harmonize the Stomach, strengthen the Spleen, tonify *qi*, nourish blood and *yin*. Lesser known functions include its ability to clear fire, useful for pathogenic heat generated through radiation and chemotherapy. It is by way of nourishing blood that ST-36 (*zu san li*) also calms the spirit.

The purpose of moxibustion for blood deficient neutropenia is to tonify and what better point than *zu san li*? There are several approaches to this treatment outlined in this section by direct and indirect formats.

---

[93] Deadman, 2007

Direct techniques must utilize a high-grade, and therefore, high-quality moxa, which are typically gold in color. As previously discussed, classical applications include the blistering or scarring method to essentially trap the heat and continue to stimulate the point long after treatment has ended. However, a few cautions must be included. First, low neutrophil levels indicate that the patient is more susceptible to infection. Using a high-quality burn cream as a base can be a useful safety measure. Its protective quality will reduce the potential for a small burn mark. In this case, the practitioner must determine the quality and strength of the patient's *qi* and blood. This discernment aligns with the medical ethic as stated in the Hippocratic text, *Epidemics, Book I*, "Practice two things in your dealings with disease: either help or do not harm the patient." The *qi* in the Stomach pulse will indicate constitutional strength or weakness. So, frequent pulse checking is a reliable treatment approach to guide protocol and determine dosage.

Typically, moxibustion treatments begin by discerning the quality of the point. In deficient patterns, there is usually a subtle indentation at ST-36 (*zu san li*). The practitioner may also assess for texture (tightness) and temperature of the skin. Direct application typically utilizes three-to-five rice grain-sized or thread moxa pieces as a starting point. For tonification, the moxa is loosely rolled into the appropriate size and individually placed on the point. The moxa is carefully lit with an incense stick, and traditionally it is left to burn entirely to the skin. This process is repeated at least three times, increasing dosage as indicated by the pulse and palpation. The heat sensations reported by the patient may vary according to their constitution. More internal cold or *yang* deficiency will require continued application, compared to *yin* deficiency with heat. Once the *qi* of the Stomach pulse becomes stronger, full and rooted, then the treatment is complete.

Another point useful for neutropenia is moxibustion on *Du*-14 (*da zhui*). This is an exceptional *yang*-focused point to circulate through cancer-management treatments as an alternative to ST-36 (*zu san li*). This method was demonstrated by a mentor and skilled oncology practitioner who applied direct, rice grain moxibustion to *Du*-14 (*da zhui*) the day before chemotherapy infusions. This optimizes the immune system to prevent neutropenia and encourage the production of white blood cells. Tonification moxa over this point is invaluable.

Our protocol is to apply three to five cones rice grain-sized moxa on *Du*-14 (*da zhui*) the day before neutrophil levels are evaluated. In many cases, the levels remain within normal range or increase. Moxa on *Du*-14 (*da zhui*) for the stated purpose is an example of accessing *yang* to treat *yin*. It is a *yang* type of treatment (fire/heat) on the *yang* aspect of the body that utilizes a point where the six *yang* meridians cross the *Du* channel. This lends to the point's ability to strongly tonify *qi* and *yang*. Since *qi* is needed to build blood, its influence with blood production attains stability.

Cancer-related Fatigue

One of the most pervasive symptoms relative to cancer is fatigue. Normal energy patterns of an individual drop and fluctuate dramatically, influenced by medications, cytotoxic therapies and radiotherapy, as well as the disease itself. Cancer related fatigue (CRF) is a condition that occurs through active treatment but can also persist for years after treatment is complete. Although CRF is an expected symptom in conventional oncology and reported by 95% of patients experiencing some form of cancer treatment.[94] Western medicine has limited means of addressing this symptom, and while patients are closely monitored, they are left to deal with it on their own.

The characteristics of CRF are myriad and non-discriminant in their presentation, affecting the physical and emotional terrain. The most obvious symptoms relate to physical energy levels. Cancer patients frequently report constant, low-grade fatigue not improved by rest or a good night's sleep. The fatigue is also unpredictable, making it difficult for patients to work, plan activities or keep appointments. Other characteristics include a feeling of heaviness throughout the body, weakness and lethargy. The fluctuations in physical energy influence emotional balance and capacity as well. When the physical self is compromised, there is a clear link to mental health and wellness. It is difficult to maintain optimism when the body is depleted, or in pain, particularly for long periods of time. Clinically, we have observed the decline of cheerful patients with positive dispositions who become withdrawn and disconnected. There is a decrease in desire

---

[94] Hofman et al., 2007

to tend to their personal appearance, and this in turn disrupts interest in social activity and engagement.

Physical and emotional fatigue over long treatment times can lead toward patterns of depression and withdrawal. Chinese medicine treatments focus on cultivating depleted energy on multiple physiological levels. The utilization of moxibustion has never been more warranted than in cancer related fatigue. The following material will provide the reader with the foundations of Chinese medicine diagnosis related to this condition. Once established, the purpose and technique of moxibustion therapy determined by clinical experience and efficacy is outlined.

Chinese Medicine Patterns

Western medicine views the body, health and disease as a mechanical system that can be evaluated and diagnosed in a reductionist manner. The linear path toward diagnosis is achieved with biopsy, imaging and analysis of tissue and blood, for example. By contrast, Chinese medicine relies upon the theory of interdependence among the organs, channels and their related patterns to create a root-branch diagnosis. However, due to the complexity of TCM oncology, a common clinical occurrence is the natural tendency to observe and focus treatment on the acute condition often to alleviate discomfort, which is a valid therapeutic approach. But, this limits the capacity of TCM therapy and aligns with the more modern medical system of reactionary care, instead of preventative.

For TCM, there are few conditions that better highlight this challenge than the issue of cancer related fatigue. In general, the TCM clinician is familiar with patients who complain of low energy; it is a pervasive ailment in this relative fast-paced world we reside in. Fatigue is characterized by either a deficient or excess condition, or more often a mixture of excess and deficiency. For example, Spleen *qi* deficiency with dampness causing low energy is a common clinical site. This kind of general fatigue is slow to improve because it requires close attention, and it is rare that patients can take a month off from work and obligations just to focus on their health. As a result, energy declines gradually, and the opportunity for illness becomes even more prominent. Chronic, persistent imbalances of the body manifest into disease becoming at its most severe form, cancer. This specific mixed diagnostic pattern is illustrated through the lens of Chinese medicine as an excess (cancer cells) and deficient (fatigue) presentation. The associated symptoms are therefore exacerbated by previous state of health, the disease itself, surgery, chemotherapy and/or radiation therapy.

The fact that TCM recognizes the significance of one's relative state of health prior to cancer diagnosis indicates why and how it can alleviate CRF, as well as other complex conditions, more effectively than other types of traditional medicine. For example, a patient undergoing multiple rounds of radiation with a constitutional tendency toward blood or *yin* deficiency will experience more pronounced excess or deficient heat symptoms due to the toxic, hot nature of radiotherapy. Further, if a person is older and generally *yang* deficient, their body's ability to endure repetitive cycles of chemotherapy is already compromised by that vacuity pattern. For a patient who has constitutionally weak Lungs, exposure to cytotoxic treatments will further devastate their *wei qi*, the energy responsible for immunity, leading to opportunistic viruses like colds and flus. The ability to ascertain previous health patterns by way of TCM principles and diagnosis is profoundly beneficial for the practitioner. It is through unfolding the layers of constitutional health that treatments are molded specifically to the individual, which make them that much more effective.

Chinese medical theory can correlate the following organ systems to cancer-related fatigue: Liver, Spleen and Stomach. The *Su Wen* Chapter 9 states that the Liver is the root of extreme fatigue.[95] The Liver stores blood and also governs and generates the sinews. Essentially, ensuring the sinews remain nourished and healthy. The sinews connect muscle to bone and thus motor function is heavily influenced by the Liver. If the Liver blood is weak, then daily activities become more difficult and stamina declines. The Liver and Kidney have the same source and so cannot be separated. Therefore, in treating one, the other is also treated. The Kidneys store *essence* and are integral to the production of blood and are responsible for will (*zhi*) and fortitude. This is clinically significant because clearly fatigue influences physical ability and strength, but it also weakens the mental and emotional capacity of a cancer patient.

The Spleen organ in Chinese medicine is essential to fundamental concepts of balance and vitality. It governs the muscles, as well as the four

---

[95] Unschuld, 2011

limbs and is the main organ that generates *qi* and blood in the body, which correlates to one's perception of energy. The Spleen also controls intellect (*yi*) and relates to thinking and concentration. Because the Spleen governs the muscles, it therefore has influence over the Liver and contributes to physical fatigue. Within this understanding, mental lethargy is likely to occur as well as a result of the Spleen's vacuity pattern.

When we speak of the Spleen, we must also think of its paired organ the Stomach, which has its own hand along with the Spleen in the production of *qi* and blood. The condition of the patient's Stomach *qi* corresponds not only to fatigue, but also to every condition or disease. The *Su Wen* Chapter 18 illustrates this concept. When the Stomach *qi* is strong, then there is a good prognosis. If the Stomach *qi* is weak, then it is a poor prognosis, and if there is no Stomach *qi*, then the condition will be fatal.[96]

Essentially, the most fundamental aspect of the treatment of cancer-related fatigue comes down to the treatment of *qi* and blood. It could be argued this is over simplistic and could be the case for every condition treated by TCM. Yes, a patient may have *yin* deficiency with empty heat or *yang* deficiency and phlegm, for example, and those should be treated. But if we fail to protect the Liver and Kidney as well as the Spleen and Stomach, the blood and *qi* become compromised. As a result, the body will take from its inherent reserves, one's *essence*. The depletion of *essence* will lead to a quicker decline in the patient's condition. Ultimately, *yin* and *yang* will separate, and death will occur. For fatigue is not just a by-product of treatment, but it is a warning that the body is struggling to deal with the disease and treatment(s). Remember the old saying in TCM: the more complex the condition the simpler the treatment.

Moxibustion for Cancer-related Fatigue
GB-39 (*Xuan Zhong*) + ST-36 (*Zu San Li*)

In our clinic, this potent point combination is used routinely and relied upon as most effective for CRF, providing deep nourishment to *qi*, blood, and marrow. For patients who are too weak or sensitive to receive acupuncture,

---

[96] Unschuld, 2011

applying moxa to these paired points addresses mild to severe vacuity patterns in both acute and chronic forms. ST-36 (*zu sanli*) generates *qi* and blood and research indicates it increases white blood cell counts. GB-39 (*xuan zhong*) is the "Influential Point of Marrow" and treats weakness and flaccidity of the limbs both deficient conditions. In addition, the function of this point lends itself to a unique bond as it connects to the Kidney, which is responsible for producing marrow. Though limited texts reference the inherent link between Gallbladder and Kidney, we find that direct or indirect moxa at this point deeply nourishes the Kidneys and improves *qi*, as well as immunity. This point combination strengthens the two main organs responsible for the production of *qi* and blood, in addition to supporting both pre-heaven and post-heaven *essence*.

The subtle nature of moxa depends on cumulative and consistent applications to warrant the most long-lasting effect. The constraints of private practice do not allow for daily moxa treatments, and as a result, we teach patients how to apply this therapy at home with a moxa stick. Beginning with the purpose of treatment, we teach them point location, observation of skin tone, color and texture, the importance of palpation to feel for heat intensity, and we recommend specific dosages and duration according to the patient's diagnosis and constitution. As an example, for a CRF condition we advise an average of five to ten minutes of indirect moxa on each point, unilaterally, once per day.

Du-4 (*Ming Men*) + Du-20 (*Bai Hui*)

The *Du* channel, also known as the Governing vessel, is one of eight extraordinary meridians and classically referred to as the 'Sea of the *Yang*.' Symptoms of CRF align uniquely with *qi-yang* deficient patterns of TCM. Classical characterization of the *Du* channel enables treatment of a myriad of conditions that affect the spinal column, urinary system, gastrointestinal tract, febrile or heat disorders, wind manifestations such as epilepsy or dizziness, as well as heart-related conditions, such as palpitations.[97] It is therefore common to needle the *Du* channel for acute symptoms as they relate to chronic disease, but it is the application of moxibustion on *Du*-4

---

[97] Deadman, 2007

(*ming men*) that we emphasize as a result of its innate ability to warm and tonify *yang*, the underlying pattern most often seen in CRF.

Its partnered point, *Du-20* (*bai hui*), is located at the apex of the head and hence the most *yang* point on the body. It is the point of the "Sea of Marrow," where all the *yang qi* of the body meet. By virtue of this location, it can raise sinking *yang qi*, as well as descend excess *yang* that has risen to the head. Classical physician, Zhu Dan-Xi notes clinical usage of three moxa cones on this point for chronic disease, *qi* deficiency and incessant diarrhea.[98] In CRF, indirect moxibustion on *bai hui* is effective not just for low energy, but for heart-related matters, when the physical lethargy influences the emotional wellness and patients express agitation, anxiety, sadness, crying or hopelessness. This correlates to the point's action of benefiting the brain and calming the spirit, noting that some classical interpretations recognize the spirit being housed in the brain, and can therefore harmonize psycho-emotional imbalances.

The unique combination of treating *Du-20* (*bai hui*) and *Du-4* (*ming men*) with moxibustion profoundly cultivates the *yang qi* and raises clear *yang* to benefit the patient both physically and mentally. In the stages of cancer, the diagnosis of *yang* deficiency is mostly present in older patients or those in the end-stage of the cancer journey when vitality is labored and depleted. Therefore, these points are clinically useful specifically for cases of cancer-related fatigue with marked *qi* and *yang* deficiency. Moxa applied to these points strengthens the *yang*, as well as the *yuan* (original) *qi* and Kidney *essence*.

Ren-4 (*Guan Yuan*) + Ren-6 (*Qi Hai*)

In contrast to harnessing the *yang* energy of the *Du* channel as discussed above, the application of moxa to the *Ren* channel is equally significant. Also referred to as the Conception vessel and one of the eight extraordinary meridians, the *Ren* meridian is profoundly *yin* in nature, originating from the uterus in females. Its pathway traverses along the anterior midline of the body, in mirrored opposition to its inseparable counterpart, *Du* channel. Of the entire *Ren* pathway, it is the lower abdomen that houses the

---

[98] Deadman, 2007.

most potent energy to nourish vitality and *essence*, precisely where *guan yuan* and *qi hai* are located. Of the hundreds of acupoints in the meridian system, these points are fundamental to the enrichment of *yin* and the Kidneys. In order to access both points with moxibustion techniques, the moxa box method of application infuses deep, nourishing heat to the *dan tian* or energy center to nourish blood, *yin* and *essence*.

The moxa box is approximately five-by-three inches, and six inches deep with a fine mesh sealed inside several inches above the skin. Coarse grain moxa is placed on the mesh and the box is sealed and placed over *Ren-4* (*guan yuan*) and *Ren-6* (*qi hai*). The patient has access to the box and can easily lift it above the umbilicus when it becomes too warm. A standard course of treatment lasts 20–30 minutes. This is another opportunity to demonstrate home-care with moxibustion if a patient has a well-ventilated area to do moxa treatment. The varying levels of fatigue and cofactors that accompany CRF are extensive, but the simple and effective application of moxa over these two acupoints is undeniably resourceful and therapeutic.

Radiation Fibrosis Syndrome

The effects of radiation can result in a condition referred to as radiation fibrosis syndrome (RFS). This is a potential complication from radiotherapy as a result of damage to blood vessels and adjacent tissue. RFS is a progressive condition that can manifest weeks and even years following conventional treatment. Any tissue type may be affected, such as skin, viscera, tendon, ligament, nerves, bones and internal organs, as a result of radiation toxicity damaging healthy cells.[99] There are a myriad of symptoms associated with this condition, but the primary complaint corresponds to limited mobility, rigidity of the musculoskeletal system specific to the area of radiation exposure, as well as localized swelling and inflammation. Once this occurs there are very limited treatment options. Physical therapy is the primary modality approved by radiation oncologists, but massage, heat therapy or myofascial release is cautioned due to the conventional understanding that local manipulation or heat application would lead to internal irritation and inflammation.

---

[99] Hojan, 2013

Chinese Medicine Patterns

This cancer-related condition is an excess condition in Chinese medicine. The toxic heat of radiotherapy causes depletion of *yin* and fluids. Subsequently, there is an effect on the nourishment of tendons, sinews and organs. Blood, as a *yin* element, is depleted and without this precious substance, the body does not receive its energy to thrive and remain supple and strong. RFS is an extension of this deficiency, characterized by multiple pathogenic factors including phlegm, heat and toxin accumulation. This results in extreme *qi* and blood stagnation impairing the smooth flow of these substances. The treatment principle addresses the excess and deficient patterns that present, dispersing the phlegm and stagnation, invigorating *qi* and blood, clearing heat, dissolving masses, nourishing blood and *yin*.

Moxibustion for Radiation Fibrosis Syndrome

Moxibustion may seem counterintuitive given that heat therapy is generally considered a contraindication with signs of heat, such as redness or swelling seen in RFS. There is a concern that its effects will inflame or worsen the condition. This is especially true with respect to philosophy and clinical application in Western medical paradigms. However, TCM relies upon the treatment philosophy of "like treats like," with proper application of moxibustion therapy. Despite the symptoms of RFS being excess in nature, our clinical experience has proven that with proper technique of hot moxa treatments, there is an immediate change in presentation, and one that becomes even more evident with repeated sessions.

This particular technique occurs with the application of larger, tightly packed moxibustion cones that facilitate a slow, longer burn time. This method generates more heat within the point or area being treated to facilitate the scattering of the heat toxin as well as to encourage *wei qi* (defensive *qi*) to the surface. Chinese medicine theory emphasizes the importance of allowing the heat to disperse through the skin by removing the cone without covering the point with the fingers to elicit a therapeutic response. However, it is crucial that the practitioner quickly place the next cone in the same location, if necessary, to maintain a steady, high level of heat. When the tissue softens and there is less firmness and density with palpation, this indicates positive change and internal heat reduction. In addition to applying pressure to assess tissue quality, the practitioner should visibly observe a decrease in localized swelling.

It is important to state that this type of technique needs to be done with the full understanding and consent of the patient, and by those practitioners who are experienced and confident with moxibustion. In a case of RFS, the integrity of the skin, sensory function, and normal sensation has been greatly compromised due to radiation therapy. By and large, Western-trained doctors believe heat is contraindicated with signs of swelling and redness, and as a result, caution patients to receive any kind of physical or manual therapy, because of the higher level of sensitivity. Thus, the practitioner needs to judge appropriate strength of treatment through their own skill and observation, without relying on the patient's feedback because they may not feel the heat as acutely.

To review, safe method and application of hot moxibustion therapy is highlighted below:

- Type: coarse, green, low-grade moxibustion to create an intense, strong *dispersing* heat
- Size: moxa is shaped into very tight, firm cones in order to create a slow, intense heat (approximately the size of a Hershey's Kiss)
- Quantity: 4–6 cones are placed directly on the specific areas with most fibrotic, tight, dense tissue
- Method: Using an incense stick, each cone is lit and watched carefully as it burns toward the skin. The cone is removed when the patient reports a sensation of heat directly under the cone, or the practitioner estimates that enough heat has accumulated locally
- Technique: The cone is removed with forceps and placed in a cup of water. The point is *not* covered by the finger to retain heat, but rather to allow the heat to disperse
- Duration: This technique is repeated on each point until there are palpatory and/or visual changes, or the practitioner deems it adequate for treatment

In summary, moxibustion is one of the oldest modalities in traditional Chinese medicine and from the perspective of archaeological evidence, certainly predates acupuncture. Its value for the practitioner lies in its versatility of administration, and its demonstrated ability to have immediate, positive, effects on how the patient feels as well as to positively influence important lab values that determine critical forms of standard care administration in cancer treatment, such as chemotherapy. For the patient, its value lies in a potent form of self-care that not only empowers the patient to have some control of their health and wellbeing but can also help them to fight some of the more intractable cancer related side effects such as fatigue and nausea. While a relatively simple and potentially powerful therapy, its long-term benefits lie in consistent administration that needs to be taught and/or administered by a licensed professional.

References

Deadman, P., & Al-Khafaji, M. (2007). *A Manual of Acupuncture* (2nd Ed.). Hove, East Sussex, England: Journal of Chinese Medicine Publications.

Hofman, M., Ryan, J., Figueroa-Moseley, C., Jean-Pierre, P., & Morrow, G. (2007). Cancer-related fatigue: The scale of the problem. *The Oncologist*. 12(1), 4–10. doi: 10.1634theoncologist.12-S1–4

Hojan, K., & Milecki, P. (2013). Opportunities for Rehabilitation of Patients with Radiation Fibrosis Syndrome. Retrieved August 24, 2018, from https://www.ncbi.nlm.nih.gov/pmc/articles/PMC4056465/

Unschuld, P. U., & Tessenow, H. Trans. (2011). Huang Di Nei Jing Su Wen. Berkeley: University of California Press.

Wang, Z., & Wang, J. (2005), *Ling Shu Acupuncture*. Anaheim, CA: Ling Shu Press.

Wheeler, J., Coppock, B., & Chen, C. (2009). Does the burning of moxa (Artemisia vulgaris) in traditional Chinese medicine constitute a health hazard? *Acupuncture in Medicine, 27*(1), 16–20. doi:10.1136/aim.2009.000422

Young, M. (2012). *The Moon Over Matsushima Insights into Moxa and Mugwort*. UK: Godiva Books.

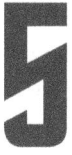

5 Chinese Herbal Medicine

"It is easy to get a thousand prescriptions but hard to get one single remedy."

Chinese Proverb

At the heart of Chinese medicine is a vast pharmacopeia. There are combinations of thousands of herbs written into classic formulations, upon which modern practitioners depend. This modality is deeply-rooted in the practice, likely because it dates back to 1066–221 B.C. where relics show illustrations of plants, case studies and described various topics of herbal properties.[100] The *Shen Nong Ben Cao Jing (Divine Husbandman's Classic of Materia Medica)* is the first text on Chinese herbal medicine. It is a compilation written by numerous scholars in 2nd century A.D. In it, 365 single herbs are examined, including dosage, temperatures, channels, indications and toxicity. Although this classical literature laid the foundation for herbal prescription, it was Li Shi-Zhen who wrote the first complete pharmacopeia, *Ben Cao Gang Mu (Compendium of Materia Medica)* in 1178 A.D.[101] Over the course of 27 years, he compiled lists of herbs, their individual properties, descriptions and illustrations of 1,892 single herbs and 11,000 formulas.[102]

For doctors of Chinese medicine, there is an intrinsic bond to plant medicinals. It's simply part of the medical lineage. As a singular modality,

---

[100] Chen et al., 2004
[101] ibid
[102] ibid

herbal therapy has stood the test of time, maintaining its presence through the course of biomedical evolution. Its fluidity, as well as complexity, is illustrated by its unique capacity to evolve alongside scientific advancements throughout medical history. It's no wonder that there is a certain enchantment when studying herbal medicine. This enthusiasm begins in introductory herb classes and follows TCM practitioners from school into private clinics, where pharmacies are built. Shelves are stocked with patent medicines, encapsulated granules, bulk raw herbs, tinctures and many other prepared forms of herbs, all ready to be prescribed accordingly. The therapeutic efficacy of herbs is so deeply ingrained, it is hard to reconcile when patients are hesitant to take herbal medicine. This is particularly true in cases of chronic or recalcitrant conditions that require a form of daily treatment, which herbs provide.

Before delving into the clinical aspects of herbal prescription for cancer, this chapter offers a brief introduction into the dynamics of herbs within science and research. To date, in the IO discipline, Chinese herbs have yet to meet the standards of evidence-based medicine (EBM), though thousands of studies are underway, which is encouraging. We analyzed an extensive array of published articles, from international research hospitals to leading cancer institutions, in order to assess the current, as well as potential role, of TCM herbs for cancer management and recovery. The clinical application of herbs for cancer management cannot be detailed enough. One chapter on the subject is merely scratching the surface of herbal integrative oncology. The skilled TCM practitioner can utilize the presented recommendations as basic frameworks but must continue to study both Chinese and Western oncology approaches.

While Chinese medicine is steadfast, as it has been for millennia, it must continue to adapt to modern medicine and this requires diligent study and research. To date, there is limited formal training on this subject in the West for TCM practitioners. While this chapter is in no way conclusive, it is designed to broaden the scope of understanding and therapeutic application of herbs for cancer patients.

Beyond learning introductory approaches to herbal oncology, it is equally important that practitioners are well-versed and prepared to engage in collaborative conversations with patients, family members and other physicians. We have committed a section of this chapter to highlight the most common questions to better prepare the TCM clinician. As with anything in the practice of Chinese medicine, learning occurs only through experience and patience, a path we continue to embark on. That is where we began many years ago, which inspired the material presented in this chapter.

Current Research and Trends of Herbal Medicine

In the West, Chinese medicine is steadily growing as a result of acupuncture therapy, which has gained recognition in mainstream health and wellness indus- tries. As a result, acupuncture represents the entirety of TCM. We are more familiarly referred to as acupuncturists, not Chinese medicine practitioners. As such, patient populations and medical professionals are familiar with only one modality in the system of TCM. The irony of this situation is that while acupuncture is profoundly effective, Chinese medicine traditionally depends on herbal prescription to address internal and complex diseases. This is even more the case in oncology where the body is routinely exposed to rather harsh and damaging forms of conventional medicine. In these treatments, herbs may be integrated to heal and rebuild as a daily form of medicine. Supplemented by acupuncture and moxibustion, the whole person is treated.

And yet, herbs are frequently the last modality to be considered and accepted. Western medical practitioners are reluctant to approve an alternative, unfamiliar treatment method that is foreign to conventional approaches. This is expected given the minimal exposure to holistic disci- plines in medical school, and more importantly, there is a significant lack of scientific literature on the subject. This creates an inherent obstacle for cancer patients seeking integrative medical care, but also limits the ways in which Chinese medicine is utilized.

Above all, the most predominant barrier to herbal prescription directly correlates to scientific merit. Are herbs an accepted form of evidence-based medicine (EBM)? This question has been and continues to be explored tirelessly. This is illustrated by the approximate 89,300 articles that examine the therapeutic potential of plant-based medicine in oncology dating back to the early 1980s.[103] Researchers analyze the molecular profile of singular

---

[103] Morelle, 2017

herbs, isolating substances that are characterized into specific anticancer functions in malignancy. Specifically, studies focus on herbal mechanisms that inhibit cellular proliferation, promote apoptosis (programmed cell death), potentiate chemotherapeutic medicine and prevent metastatic spread.

For example, Chinese herbs that invigorate the blood actively promote and maintain healthy circulation in the vessels to prevent blood stasis patterns. The herb, *dan shen* (salvia miltiorrhiza), demonstrates this action and is widely used in herbal formulas for cancer. A recent study explored its potential anticancer effects in high-quality randomized controlled trials (RCT). Researchers isolated the bioactive components responsible for inhibiting the migration, or invasion of metastatic cancer cells, and found this herb triggered apoptosis as an anti-inflammatory agent.[104] In essence, the mechanism of action works in a manner that potentiates the effects of conventional methods such as chemotherapeutic agents by destroying tumor cells.

Although there are thousands of international studies about herbal medicine, scientific methodology is not always consistent. For example, RCTs on herbal medicine between 1966–2003 published in Medline largely yielded incomplete findings due to allocation concealment, inadequate controls, minimal blinding and intention-to-treat analyses.[105] As a consequence, these studies are not well-substantiated, which renders them useless as means to illustrate the efficacy of phytochemicals. Other systematic reviews that analyze non-clinical *in vivo* or *in vitro* studies demonstrate questionable study protocols and data reporting, again impacting the way in which herbs are accepted in allopathic medicine.[106] The end result indicated by the current contention over Chinese herbs for cancer is that they do not yet qualify as a form of EBM.

Beyond the scientific reports and data, however, it is apparent that herbal medicine is on the rise. Its overall growth is illustrated by a 2013 report that found consumers in the United States spent approximately six billion dollars on herbs to maintain or improve health.[107] A 2017 study in the United States revealed that out of 26,157 respondents, 35% took

---

[104] Tianqi et al., 2019
[105] Gagnier et al., 2006
[106] ibid
[107] Rashrash et al., 2017

one herbal product daily, while most took three.[108] Within this statistic, 43% used herbs for cancer and its related conditions.[109] Thus, there is an undeniable movement toward natural medicine therapies. We observe this energy in general practice, as patients consciously choose holistic remedies in lieu of over the counter medications or pharmaceuticals to treat acute or chronic conditions. This is likely related to a growing discontent and awareness that standard Western medicine is reactionary. Disease is treated only after confirmed illness or diagnosis, and treatment recourse relies on pharmaceuticals that are often accompanied by a host of side-effects. This is a phenomenal paradigm shift in healthcare, specifically because we can track the evolution of integrative medicine largely to individuals who sought alternative means of healing, venturing outside the established medical norms.

It's particularly perplexing that TCM herbs, as well as most botanicals, are so highly cautioned because the composition of many prescription drugs are derived from plant-based materials. An analysis of natural products identified as sources of synthetic compounds from 1982–2002, determined that an average of 62% of non-synthetic chemicals stem from small, molecular components of plant products.[110] A significant example of this is the antiestrogen drug prescribed in hormone positive breast cancer, Tamoxifen. This hormone therapy was developed from a 1962 discovery that identified bark on the Pacific yew tree (taxus brevifolia) contained cytotoxic effects with active molecules.[111] Further characterization of the molecular profile demonstrated that the microtubules were stabilized within the cell, and this prevented breakdown that enabled normal mitosis, ultimately impeding cancer cell replication.[112] As a result, massive amounts of Pacific yew trees were razed to extract the bark. Approximately three mature trees were required for one cancer patient.[113] This environmental impact led the pharmaceutical company that acquired

---

[108] ibid
[109] ibid
[110] Newman et al., 2003
[111] Bryan, 2011
[112] Schiff et al., 1980
[113] Bryan, 2011

the licensing from the National Cancer Institute (NCI), Bristol-Meyer Squibb, to examine other approaches in the production of this drug. Accordingly, plant cell fermentation shifted methods of production and overharvesting of the yew tree.

Much of this tenuous dynamic is influenced by pharmaceutical companies whose primary focus is patenting for profit. Opponents and skeptics to herbal medicine often cite a "lack of research" as a reason to prohibit or avoid using herbal medicine. Never mind that there are conservatively hundreds of herbs which have been taken for thousands of years as first forms of medicine. Not to mention Chinese herbal medicine has been practiced alongside Western medicine for over 50 years in Asia. Other than the educational and cultural biases that exist toward natural medicine, especially herbal therapies, probably the biggest roadblock to herbal medicine's continued evolution and integration with Western medicine relates to economics.

Pharmaceutical companies often cite the expense involved in research as well as supplying products in the market. Another interpretation of this reasoning recognizes the difficulty in patenting herbal compounds. Pharmaceutical companies are mainly interested in creating or discovering new active ingredients because these are patentable. With at least an estimated 390,000 species of plants on the planet, and thousands being discovered every year, it is possible that new, singularly definable ingredients exist, but again the cost of research comes in to play.[114] Big pharma can get around the issue of patenting known active ingredients by creating a unique method to extract or augment a key ingredient, but it is usually only a matter of time before competitors figure out their own method or a workaround. This is illustrated in the previous discussion on Tamoxifen and the yew tree.

The structure itself, including cost, rules, volume and length, of accepted research in the West largely makes it prohibitive towards anyone but large companies and institutions to undertake. So, instead of having doctors, healthcare practitioners and researchers leading the way and providing direction on healthcare, it is led by profit. Moreover, funding for research in order to receive Federal Drug Administration (FDA) approval is hard to

---

[114] Morelle, 2016

come by. For example, evaluation of aqueous extracts of the Chinese herb *ban zhi lian* (scutellaria barbata) were studied as a potential oral therapy in the treatment of metastatic breast cancer under FDA Investigational New Drug License (IND).[115] In the materia medica, *ban zhi lian* (scutellaria barbata) as a singular herb functions to clear heat, eliminate toxin, invigorate blood and stop bleeding. With respect to cancer, it is also considered an antineoplastic herb that targets tumors of the lung and gastrointestinal system. *Ban zhi lian* (scutellaria barbata) also prevents recurrence, indicated by a report that found a dose-dependent effect in promoting macrophage function *in vitro*, as well as tumor inhibition *in vivo*.[116]

This herb was studied in two clinical trials for cases of advanced breast cancer. The participants had expected survival rates of 3–4 months and had completed an average of 3.9 conventional method treatments prior to the study. Phase I clinical trials demonstrated a reduction in tumor size, delays in disease progression and improved survival slightly past 11 months.[117] This study elucidated the mechanistic action of *ban zhi lian* (scutellaria barbata) and characterized its active ingredients. Positive results indicated inhibition of breast cancer cells by inducing apoptosis, programmed cell death.[118] Despite these findings, further funding was not approved for Phase II clinical trials, illustrating the complexity of science, funding and ultimately, profit.

Singular components of plant material, such as scutellaria barbata, are often studied individually to determine active ingredients, but reports are underway that analyze combinations of herbs for cancer treatment. This relates to the synergy that occurs when single herbs are combined in formulas to balance and potentiate effects. Researchers at the University of Adelaide are studying *ku shen* (radix sophorae flavescentis) injection (CKI), a tumor fighting compound consisting of *ku shen* (radix sophorae flavescentis) and *bai tu ling* (rhizoma smilacis glabrae) used in China as an adjunct to standard chemotherapy. This is referred to as a systems biology approach. Interestingly, it aligns with Chinese medicine's understanding that synergism among multiple modalities or substances yields greater

---

[115] Rugo et al., 2006
[116] Wong et al., 1996
[117] Cohen, 2015
[118] ibid

outcomes, as parts to a greater whole. The researchers examined breast cancer cells grown in the laboratory and utilized technology that enabled identification of genes and pathways. When targeted by CKI injections, the regulation of the cell cycle is altered in such a way that the cancer cells are eradicated.[119] This process considers all measurable facets, the system wide molecular mechanism, when analyzing complex biological systems and not just a sole variable.

As it stands, there are few examples of Chinese herb derived drugs. An example of the potential of herbal therapy in modern medicine is the semi-synthetic drug Artemisinin, which is derived from the TCM herb *qing hao* (artemisia annua). It is the leading drug in the treatment of malaria used to save millions of lives since its development. It was discovered by Professor YouYou Tu in the early 1970s in response to a directive from Mao Tse-tung to cure malaria. Politics aside, this exemplifies the reality that herbs are innately medicinal, and when health is prioritized above patents and profit, real advancements in curing chronic disease is possible.

Herbal medicine is deeply embedded throughout Asian countries, including Japan, Korea and China for longevity, health and wellness. It is not just thousands of years of empirical research that illustrates this point, but through its presence in modern practice where Chinese medicine practitioners work alongside their Western trained colleagues. It truly encompasses the best of the old, with the best of the new, and already demonstrates legitimate integrative oncology. Western-trained physicians in China are taught Chinese medicine approaches, in order to make suitable recommendations for shared patients. This collaborative effort recognizes the value of both disciplines: one that can interface head-on with neoplastic disease, supported by the other which limits physiological harm in the process.

These approaches are evident in cancer hospitals in China that not only prescribe herbal medicine but administer it intravenously. For example, intramuscular injections of *huang qi* (radix astragali) are given prior to surgery to protect the immune system. The biochemical mechanism of *huang qi* raises white blood cells (WBC) in peripheral blood and elevates t-lymphocytic activity.[120] This application strengthens the immune system

---

[119] Science Daily, 2016
[120] Peiwen, 2003

in order to prevent neutropenic conditions during post-surgical recovery, and in doing so, limits harm and expedites healing. This reflects a primary principle in a comprehensive system of cancer treatment, referred to as *Fu Zheng* therapy or "Support Vital Qi." In terms of integration, *Fu Zheng* represents the whole organism in relation to disease and serves as an instrumental guide for TCM herbalists.

The Integration

In the practice of Chinese medicine, practitioners observe physical presentations as a result of internal disharmony. Diagnostic patterns and principles are established, before any modality is applied therapeutically. These concepts are ingrained in every clinical technique from acupuncture to moxibustion, as demonstrated in previous chapters. The difference between these modalities and herbal medicine, is that they are a form of external treatment. In turn, they equate with relative safety and a certain degree of effectiveness that can be measured almost immediately, with little to no side effects, or risk. Herbs, however, once consumed cannot be as easily or quickly measured by imaging or labs. Instead, the response is subjective, causing a relative unknown as to measured internal effects. This causes varying degrees of concern in Western medicine contexts because of potential, unforeseen interactions with allopathic treatment plans. And this concern should not be ignored in integrative oncology systems, nor by the TCM profession.

Chinese herbal therapy is uniquely suited for IO because it treats the whole person. It is in essence patient-centered. Singular herbs are combined into formulas to have a direct therapeutic effect in very specific degrees, from addressing acute symptoms, to the underlying cause of disease. For example, singular herbs enhance the immune system, such *huang qi* (radix astragali), but in combination with *bai zhu* (atractylodes) and *fang feng* (radix saposhnikovia) their immune strengthening effects are amplified by their synergistic relationship. Further, their interaction occurs by virtue of their ability to protect the body from pathogens entering the system, thus acting as agents that prevent further injury to the body. In Western terms, the mechanism of action by herbal formulas are multifaceted. They potentiate the rate of phagocytosis, the process by which pathogens and cell debris are removed. In addition, they promote antibody formation, lengthen the survival of antibodies and prevent leukopenia.[121] Ultimately, herbal therapy is integrative and dual-focused: eradicate the excess pathogenic factor (cancerous cells) and fortify the constitutional terrain.

There are two primary goals when prescribing herbs for a cancer patient. First, to protect the patient from physical decline due to disease or medical intervention. In our clinic, this is the first message shared in intake. If the patient becomes too weak, malnourished, depressed or suffers inordinate complications causing a delay in chemotherapy or radiation, the cancer is left untreated. Herbs rectify imbalances that weaken the body. Second, herbal medicine considers the root and addresses any imbalance of vital substances that constitute one's health. This includes qi, blood, jing (essence), body fluids and shen (spirit), so that the body heals as a whole, whether from cancer or related conditions. With this principle in mind, herbal formulations optimize physiological performance when impacted by cytotoxic agents, radiation or surgical procedures. This aligns with antineoplastic principles, further outlined in the following ways:

- Enhance quality of life: alleviate physical and emotional side effects
- Boost the immune system: maintain white blood cells, prevent leukopenia
- Maintain circulation of qi and blood, optimize healthy blood flow
- Nourish yin of Liver and Kidney, generate fluids
- Regulate digestion by tonifying Spleen and Stomach
- Prevent metastatic spread, anticancer
- Resolve toxins, and alleviate pain

Writing an herbal prescription is a process that brings the scientific and artistic side of Chinese medicine into play. No two practitioners will write the same prescription, matching ingredients and dosages. Completed formulations reflect the skill of the practitioner and breadth of knowledge on the subject

---

[121] Lahans, 2007

matter it is designed to treat. In TCM, pattern differentiation generates an established set of therapeutic principles that guide the treatment plan. This is a reliable foundation upon which herbal prescription for cancer management begins. It also reflects the primary schools of thought in the treatment of neo-plastic disease. These correlate to the causative factors of tumor formation previously established: *qi* stagnation and blood stasis, damp-phlegm accumu-lation, heat toxin and *zang-fu* deficiencies.[122] Herbs are then selected based on the relative degree of excess pattern etiology versus deficiency. There is always some degree of deficiency in cancer diagnosis, whether preceding the condition or as a result of it. The application of *Fu Zheng* therapy is essential in any case to restore vital *qi*, and encourage restorative wellness to the body's terrain. In Chinese medicine this invokes the fundamental concept of balance between *yin* and *yang*, from which health derives.

The application of each and every modality in TCM reflects this inher-ent principle. The advantage of herbal prescription is its far-reaching abilities that balance disharmonies in the body routinely and cumulatively. As we tell our patients, herbs are a form of daily treatment. This is a unique benefit when it comes to herbs for malignancy because of its targeted approach. Herbs can therefore be dosed, scheduled and taken by the patient at specific times to optimize a therapeutic outcome. This is illustrated by strategies to lessen cancer-related fatigue during chemotherapy cycles, reduce heat and inflammation from radiation, or to fortify the immune system and prevent leukopenia pre- or post-surgery.

This whole-body, systemic approach considers the constitution, present pathology and potential injury from disease or medical interven-tions. Herbal formulas can therefore be effective participants along the continuum of care. Therapeutic delivery is achieved by considering three core components, which are present in any phase of cancer management:

- Constitutional patterns and physiology separate from neoplastic diagnosis
- Determining the root and branch Chinese medical diagnosis
- Assess and predict the degree of injury from conventional therapies

---

[122] Peiwen, 2003

This approach aims to attune the physiological body with necessary interventions, such as cytotoxic therapy, radiation or surgery. By doing so, the whole person can be treated. Further, this approach reflects the anti-neoplastic potential of herbal medicine. When we are asked by patients or doctors if there is risk of interaction, we explain the mechanism behind herbal integration. Chinese medicine does not utilize harsh expellants as a singular approach to aggressively eradicate malignancy. Instead, herbs facilitate innate healing capacity of the patient. In doing so, the patient has a unique window of opportunity to rebuild through each phase of conventional care, thus allowing them to complete the prescribed conventional program.

Chemotherapy

In order to select herbs that provide adjunctive care during chemotherapy, it is important that practitioners are familiar with the class of cytotoxic drugs commonly used for malignancies. This knowledge informs the integrative approach. For example, prescribing herbs according to the nadir of the chemotherapy cycle to aptly restore the body, or recognizing platinum-based agents that induce peripheral neuropathy. By understanding the differences among conventional therapies, it enables the TCM practitioner to ascertain the severity of the disease based on the oncologist's treatment plan. So, even if there is a lack of collaborative care, or the patient just hands over their chemotherapy schedule, it is possible to effectively integrate care to improve outcomes. Chemotherapeutic agents differ in terms of mechanism of action, but the end goal is shared: stop tumor cells from dividing.

While quite extensive and rapidly changing, there are commonly used antitumor drugs. For example, alkylating agents are the earliest forms of cancer treatment, dating back to the 1940s. Cancer cells are affected by damaged DNA. When alkylating agents disrupt the structure of a DNA molecule, it prevents cancer cells from multiplying, thus causing cell death. Cyclophosphamide is one of the many drugs in this class, as well as a sub-category of platinum-based compounds like cisplatin or carboplatin. Further categories of chemotherapeutic agents include, antitumor antibiotics, antimetabolites and topoisomerase inhibitors. Interestingly, a number of chemotherapeutic substances are comprised of alkaloids that are derived from certain parts of a plant, termed plant alkaloids. For example, taxanes from the Pacific yew tree (taxus), and the chemical constituents of the periwinkle plant (catharanthus rosea) comprise vinca alkaloids like vincristine. Podophyllotoxins, such as etoposide used for cancer of the uterus, lung and stomach, as well as lymphomas, are derived from the May apple plant.

Hormonal therapies are not considered chemotherapy agents but endocrine agents. Their mechanism of action is directed toward tissue that reacts to other hormonal substances. Prednisone is the most well-known example of a type of endocrine therapy. In hormone positive cancers, like breast or prostate, the use of antihormone therapies are employed to interfere with the cellular proliferation of the cancer cells.[123] Tamoxifen, previously mentioned, is an example of antiestrogen therapy, which is typically prescribed for longer duration of 5–7 years for women with estrogen positive breast cancer. Whether chemotherapy or hormone therapy, there is a range of concurrent issues that impact quality of life. Herbal formulas can therefore be extremely supportive as an element of adjunctive care.

This is achieved by timing and tailoring the herbal prescription according to the patient's chemotherapy cycles and Chinese medicine diagnosis. The dosing of each regimen is scheduled in order to maximize the eradication of cancer cells, followed by a period of recovery when the hematopoietic cells of the bone marrow can regenerate. There are cycles that occur in dose dense regimens which delivers lower dose chemotherapy on a weekly or bi-weekly basis. Other delivery means occur via an infusion pump that the patient wears for 24 hours. The initial post-chemo phase causes the most acute side effects. Often this lasts up to six days, with nausea, vomiting, fatigue, low appetite, insomnia, pain, diarrhea, anxiety and overall discomfort. While there are a myriad of herbs in the pharmacopeia that address these symptoms, we find that patients are less able to take formulas during this time, particularly when there is nausea or low appetite. Once the cytotoxic effects diminish, herbal integration is more likely. Until then, acupuncture and moxibustion are extremely effective.

Patients often report measurable difference in acute side-effects once the body metabolizes the chemotherapy. There is substantial relief, and it is often quite palpable. At this period, between infusions, the opportunity

---

[123] Lahans, 2007

to strengthen the Spleen and Stomach is maximized. The energetics of chemotherapeutic drugs, which target toxic-heat, damp-heat and phlegm are extremely cold in nature. These cold substances deplete the *qi* of the Spleen and Stomach, which further degrade the integrity of the digestive system. With this in mind, the treatment goal is to tonify and rehabilitate the gastrointestinal (GI) system as much as possible before the next infusion. This nourishes the same meridians responsible for generating blood, which protects the skin and mucosal lining of the GI tract from mouth to bowels.

Once the physiological reactions post-infusion subside, the patient is more stable. This of course depends on the stage and phase of their cancer journey, but more often that not, there is a reprieve from conventional therapies. Whether it lasts three days or three weeks, it is a period of restorative care. The goal of herbal formulas is to provide this restoration and tonify vital substances, promote bone marrow production, facilitate regulation of the circulatory, lymphatic, digestive and immune system. We often remind patients that although they feel incrementally better, their body is still reacting and recovering from the infusion. This often correlates with the nadir, when the damage to the system has caused absolute decline demonstrated by low blood chemistry values, often white blood cells and platelets. Risk of infection is at its highest, because the defensive *qi* of the body is compromised.

The third phase that occurs following the acute cytotoxic activity and the restorative stage is regenerative and preventative. The timing of chemotherapy regimens vary, but regardless, the 5–7 days before the next dose is prime opportunity for optimizing the body's resilience both physically and emotionally. The physical reminders that constantly remind the individual of their diagnosis have quieted, and in that calm, there is a mental shift that often plays out. Anticipatory nausea, increasing anxiety, worry, and insomnia begin to surface in anticipation of the next cycle. The relief of enduring another chemotherapy passes, but emotional disturbances appear. Singular herbs soften this response, and quell some degree of anxiousness that naturally accompanies the entire cancer experience.

Here we demonstrate an ebb and flow of symptoms that frequently arise in chemotherapy cycles. From the acute, to moderate stability, to the emotional terrain, it requires a great amount of endurance, stamina and support. Chinese herbal medicine can therefore move through these phases and cycles, working alongside the toxicity to potentiate the medicine's effectiveness, moderate the physical side effects, and then rebuild the body to increase its capacity to remain steadfast in all parameters of the whole person. In the following section, several cases will outline this path, illustrating the goal and function of herbal medicine in varying stages of cancer, as well as specific cancer-related conditions.

Case Study

Herbal integration for leukopenia

We began treating Cynthia, a retired high school principal at the time of her third recurrence of non-Hodgkin lymphoma (NHL), a subtype of lymphoma and blood cancer. Her initial diagnosis occurred 12 years prior when a swollen lymph node appeared in her groin, accompanied by fever, night sweats and fatigue, classic signs of NHL. This type of cancer develops when mutations occur in lymph nodes among three types of lymphocytes: B lymphocytes (B cells), responsible for producing antibodies to prevent infections, or T lymphocytes (T cells), that assist B-cells among other functions, and finally natural killer (NK) cells that act on viruses or tumors within cells. Approximately 85–90% of cases begin as B cells, which was true of Cynthia's case.[124] NHL can be further subdivided into two types: indolent (slow-growing) or aggressive (fast-growing). Cynthia was diagnosed with B-cell, indolent type and treated with a course of radiation and standard chemotherapy referred to as CHOP (cyclophosphamide, vincristine, prednisone, bleomycin).

Cynthia was familiar with Chinese medicine, having received acupuncture throughout adulthood for a variety of ailments. Despite the cancer diagnosis, she maintained good health. An active hiker who loved the outdoors, she was committed to a healthy lifestyle. An increase in fatigue and shortness of breath lead her back to the doctor who confirmed the recurrence with metastasis to the bone marrow considered stage IV. She began a regimen that consisted of bendamustine and rituximab (BR), a targeted form of cancer therapy for six cycles. The infusions were administered

---

[124] https://www.lls.org/lymphoma/non-hodgkin-lymphoma

in a two-day period, with a four-week break in between. Bendamustine is an alkylating antineoplastic agent that treats NHL. In combination with rituximab, which is an antibody therapy, they help the immune system to fight cancer cells.

Cynthia's return to complementary medicine was to address low white blood cells (WBC), a form of leukopenia. The first chemotherapy cycle caused a significant drop in absolute neutrophil counts (ANC) . The standard range is 2.1–7.7 K/uL. At the time of treatment, approximately three weeks after the first infusion, her ANC was 1.5 K/uL, even after a five-day dose of neupogen injections. Knowing her oncologist would postpone infusions if her levels continued to decline, she sought out Chinese medicine. The initial treatment aligned with the third phase, post-infusion where rebuilding and regenerating is the goal. Reluctant to try herbal prescription, she received acupuncture and moxibustion weekly to tonify blood, spleen *qi* and kidney *yang*. In addition, she was prescribed daily rounds of moxa therapy on ST-36 (*zu san li*) and GB-39 (*xuan zhong*) to further strengthen the root. Within three months, Cynthia's routine was established. Daily self-care consisted of moxa, several cups of homemade bone broth, 30 minutes of walking and *Qigong*.

Her average ANC remained around 1.4 K/uL, closely monitored by her oncologist. Chemotherapy would be postponed if pre-chemo levels dropped below 1.0 K/uL. Her physical terrain mirrored the lab measurement as well. The five-day period after chemotherapy triggered low appetite, constipation, mouth and tongue sores and bone pain from the neupogen injections. By week two, energy increased, appetite returned, and she reported, "I feel like I rebound much faster than previous chemo cycles, and that's encouraging." This continued for an additional two cycles, until a pre-chemo lab count indicated her levels were 0.7 K/uL. Chemotherapy was postponed by her oncologist who recommended a three month break for counts to increase. Essentially, monitor, watch and wait. At the point, Cynthia suddenly became curious about Chinese herbs.

The following formula was created by Chinese medicine doctor and researcher, Dr. Isaac Cohen, in cases of neutropenia. Simple, yet enormously therapeutic, it consists of four herbs: *huang qi* (radix astragali), *bai mu er* (tremella fuciformis), *ku shen* (sophora flavescens), and *ji xue teng* (caulis spatholobi). The first, *huang qi* (radix astragali), has been extensively studied for its immune enhancing enhancing effects and ability to lessen side-effects from chemotherapy, such as neurotoxicity. A meta-analysis of 1,305 relevant publications examining randomized trials with 2,815 human subjects, reported that the delivery of astragalus alongside platinum-based chemotherapy increased its effectiveness, survival, tumor response, and stimulates natural killer cell activity.[125] *Bai mu er* (tremella fuciformis) is a mushroom that nourishes yin and generates body fluids, studies indicate it also has antitumor properties; *ku shen* (sophora flavescens) clears heat and relieves toxicity. The primary alkaloid present in sophora flavescens shows potential antitumor effects in multiple types of cancers. *Ji xue teng* (caulis spatholobi) nourishes blood and is also classically considered a revitalizing herb. As previously discussed, while the singular functions of herbs are recognized for their therapeutic function, it is the synergy of ingredients that delivers higher potency and efficacy.

Cynthia integrated this formula into her daily routine and continued weekly acupuncture. Monthly lab tests allowed us to monitor changes in her values, to which we observed incremental progress. Within one month, counts increased from 0.7 K/uL to 0.8 K/uL, one month later another increase to 0.9 K/uL. The goal was to reach 1.0 K/uL before continuing chemotherapy. Thus, she was tracking very carefully and each month declared with excitement that her body was responding well, and the labs proved it. By the third month, the cumulative effect of the herbal formula catapulted her levels from 0.9 K/uL to 1.3 K/uL. This of course was not the sole contribution of the herbs, but illustrates how this added modality optimized her body's healing capacity. Her levels further increased to 1.9 K/uL, as did her energy and overall well-being. This positive change in labs increased her optimism, as well as her interaction with her recurrence, "I decided to stop worrying about cancer all the time and focus on my true-self and healing." Cynthia was able to complete her chemotherapy regimen and remained on the herbs throughout her course of care.

Neutropenia Base Formula[126]

---

huang qi (radix astragali) — 10 g
bai mu er (tremella fuciformis) — 10 g
ku shen (sophora flavescens) — 15 g
ji xue teng (caulis spatholobi) — 8 g

---

[125] McCulloch and See, 2006
[126] Cohen, 2015

In addition to writing prescriptions that target specific conditions or outcomes, as demonstrated above, herbal formulas can be dosed according to predetermined chemotherapy or radiation cycles, as well as pre or post-surgical. This is particularly beneficial when patients are concerned about adverse interactions, or for the newer TCM practitioner unfamiliar with herbal oncology. This is the opportunity to integrate *fu zheng* formulas that emphasize the individual's normal *qi* without directly interfacing with conventional protocols. However, before any prescription is issued, TCM practitioners must consider more than Chinese medicinals and their mechanism of action. An equal understanding and awareness of Western diagnostics and protocols is necessary in any form of adjunctive care. This is when the value of integrative oncology is realized both between Chinese medicine practitioners and patients but also with oncologists. Establishing rapport and trust is integral to this modality.

The framework for tailoring the delivery of herbal medicine in cancer management is multifold. It depends on the clinical experience of the practitioner, relative to patient constitution and disease severity. A clinical rule of thumb is to utilize *fu zheng* therapy as a baseline. Incorporate herbs to support vital *qi* and mitigate specific side effects in between chemotherapy cycles. This can be as simple as cumulative dosing singular herbs that enhance the immune system and vital *qi*, like *dong chong xia cao* (cordyceps), or *ren shen* (ginseng). Similarly, incorporating classic formulas to protect the Spleen and Stomach from impending injury due to cold, toxic nature of chemo agents. *Si Jun Zi Tang* (Four Gentlemen Decoction), *Shi Quan Da Bu Tang* (All Inclusive Great Tonifying Decoction), or *Ba Zhen Tang* (Eight Treasures Decoction) are appropriate for this method of application. Often we recommend patients start by integrating formulas for a period of 3–5 days, before or after an infusion. Prescribe the final dose 24 hours before scheduled infusion, and begin 48–72 hours after. This will always be dependent on how their medicine is administered and in the timing of the chemo regimen.

We highly encourage newer practitioners to start with classic formulas without modifications. Become familiar with the multitude of chemo schedules, follow the patient's progress and closely observe the ebb and flow of recovery phases. Slowly integrating classic TCM formulas illustrates an informative baseline of the potency and effectiveness of herbal medicine for cancer. This occurs without impacting the conventional protocol. Once established, practitioners can use this breadth of knowledge to modify prescriptions with more specificity.

For example, we recently provided adjunctive care for a 58-year-old male patient with stage 1B liver cancer. He was prescribed six rounds of chemotherapy, gemcitabine (antimetabolite, nadir 10–14 days) and paclitaxel protein-bound (antineoplastic, plant alkaloid). The chemo regimen was scheduled two weeks in a row, one week off. He complained of acute symptoms the night after chemo, including insomnia (due to steroid), night sweats (damp heat), and no appetite (spleen deficiency). Secondary symptoms followed days 2–5. He predominantly experienced fatigue in the afternoon with brain fog, thirst and mild abdominal distension. Neuropathy mildly affected the bottom of his feet and fingertips. His bowel movements tended toward constipation, a result of anti-nausea medications. Physical examination indicated lower leg edema. His tongue is pale, enlarged with a damp coat. Pulse is soggy and thin. At the root of this patient's presentation is Spleen *qi* deficiency.

The base herbal formula is *Liu Jun Zi Tang* (Six Gentlemen Formula) which classically treats Spleen depletion patterns with damp or phlegm. Classically, it is comprised of six herbs: *ren shen* (radix ginseng), *zhi gan cao* (glycyrrhizae radix), *fu ling* (poria), *bai zhu* (atractylodes macrocephala), *chen pi* (pericarpium citri reticulatae) and *ban xia* (pinellia rhizome). Numerous studies have demonstrated this formula's efficacy in relation to gastrointestinal issues as a result of cytotoxic therapy causing digestive injury. A recent scientific study examined the protective actions of *Liu Jun Zi Tang* (Six Gentlemen Decoction) on chemotherapy-induced neuropathy associated with cisplatin, indicating promising results.[127]

As the foundation formula, it focuses on the main TCM treatment principle: tonify Spleen *qi* and resolve damp. Secondary herbs were selected to potentiate the primary ingredients by nourishing *yin*, clearing heat-toxin, resolving phlegm, and tonifying Kidneys. The mechanism of action by the herbs, in relation to the chemotherapy and tumor, are noted below. Granulated herbs were dosed at 12 grams per day. Note that generally dosages in cancer management are upwards of 18 grams per day,

---

[127] Chiou et al., 2013

twice the normal adult dose.[128] The purpose is to generate higher levels of phytochemicals that circulate within the bloodstream.[129] In this case, the goal of herbal prescription was to lessen the severity of cytotoxic injury, alleviate symptoms and restore the body during the recovery phase in preparation for the next infusion.

Liu Jun Zi Tang (Six Gentlemen Formula) 60 g	Tonify spleen, resolve damp, metabolizes antineoplastics, prevents neurotoxicity
zhe bei mu (fritillaria thunbergii) 10 g	Clear heat, dissolve nodules, antineoplastic
mo yao (myrrha), *chi shao* 15 g (paeoniae radix rubra), *dan shen* (salviae miltiorrhizae)	Blood invigorating, compromises tumor integrity
mai men dong (ophiopogonis radix), 15 g *bai shao* (paeoniae radix alba), *shu di huang* (rehmanniae radix)	Nourish yin, protective
chuan lian zi (toosendan fructus) 15 g	Clear heat, dry damp, alleviates flank pain
xian he cao 15 g	Cools blood, stops bleeding
zhu ling 15 g	Drains damp, antineoplastic, increases white blood cells
ze xie 15 g	Drains damp, promotes urination
gan cao, sheng jiang 6 g	Harmonizes digestive integration

This herbal prescription was integrated after the patient's second round of chemotherapy. It was implemented alongside weekly acupuncture, moxibustion and nutritional recommendations to which he reported sustained appetite, energy and digestion. His pre-chemo labs also remained within normal ranges, allowing him to continue the course of chemotherapy without interruption. In addition, he incorporated physical exercise twice per week and felt well enough to return to work part-time.

Radiation

Unlike chemotherapy, radiation has less systemic effect. Ionizing radiation (IR) is targeted toward specific areas of the body, directed at solid tumors, residual tumor cells, as well as in some blood and lymph cancers. This

---

[128] Lahans, 2007

[129] ibid

lends some benefit to the patient as the side-effects are often localized to areas of exposure. Most clinical presentations include forms of skin and tissue irritation, such redness, blistering, peeling, itching, and underlying fibrosis. Radiation to the abdominal region will cause a disruption in bowel movements, mostly diarrhea. Hematopoietic function is compromised in some cases with a decline in WBC, red blood cells (RBC) or platelets for several days. Clinically, TCM treats both superficial and visible side effects but also injury to the *qi*, blood and *shen* (spirit). This often manifests as fatigue, irregular sleep patterns and mood instability. These symptoms are less likely to be shared by radiation oncologists. There tends to be a great deal of focus on the local inflammatory response and how to best alleviate skin-related issues. But there is a remarkable influence over the patient's mental-emotional wellness, addressed by herbal therapy.

In TCM, radiation is excess, pathogenic heat. This burns the *yin* of the body, causes dryness and impairs the vital *qi*. The Spleen is further injured by this process, inhibiting the production of blood that nourishes tissue, skin and hair. Similar to chemotherapy, radiation is also cycled in varying degrees. Often it is prescribed in five-week durations on a daily basis. This causes acute symptoms that affect quality of life. So, the aim is to lessen discomfort and prevent further damage. For example, we recently treated a 52-year-old woman diagnosed with stage 1A breast cancer, estrogen/progesterone (ER/PR) positive. Kathy found a lump during self-breast exam. She underwent lymph node biopsy, lumpectomy with surgical resection. Radiation was prescribed for five weeks to target the localized site of the resected tumor and adjacent lymph nodes.

The process of prescribing herbal formulas during radiation focuses less on cyclical dosing as demonstrated during chemotherapy regimens and more on reducing cumulative harm. Thus, the action of the selected herbs is primarily protective. Researchers have identified how certain phytochemicals are effective as adjunctive therapy, contrary to the concern that antioxidants interfere with radiation's maximum effect. However, *in vitro* and *in vivo* studies indicate that herbal compounds improve outcomes of radiotherapy, enhancing anticancer functions.[130] Specifically, the classic formula *Gui Pi Tang* (Restore the Spleen Decoction) has been shown to

---

[130] Jia et al., 2013

increase cellular immunocompetence when affected by IR, signaling an ability to optimize hematopoietic recovery.[131]

This study's findings correlates with the function of the formula to tonify Spleen, nourish blood and calm the spirit. In the case above, the patient's TCM diagnosis reflected many years of high stress, overwork and worry: Liver *qi* stagnation, Liver and Kidney *yin* deficiency with heat. The treatment principle was to smooth Liver *qi*, nourish *yin* and blood and clear deficient heat. The therapeutic approach in early stage presentations is to emphasize the *fu zheng* therapy principle and cultivate the root. The pathogenic factor is relatively weak, so the focus is on strengthening immunity. This is important in post-surgical cases, since surgery is a causative factor in blood and *qi* deficiency. The local trauma also causes swelling that creates fluid accumulation and blood stasis. Acupuncture and moxa addressed these acute side-effects and facilitated rapid healing with no complications.

The Chinese herbs interface with post-surgical recovery, the pathogen (residual tumor cells), and protect the terrain from impending injury caused by IR. Kathy experienced mild pre-menopausal symptoms with night sweats, agitation, vaginal dryness, anxiety and insomnia but still maintained a monthly cycle. In this case, *Liu Wei Di Huang Wan* (Six Ingredient Pill), was chosen as the base formula since it is known to reduce estrogen levels in pre-menopausal women.[132] Additional herbs were added with the following therapeutic goals, listed in the box below. Dosage was prescribed at 9 grams, twice per day.

Kathy was extremely compliant with her herbal prescription and completed her radiation therapy without complications. The most severe side-effect was local erythema and mild blistering of her skin. Local application of pure aloe vera gel and *Chin Wan Hung* burn cream alleviated the discomfort and within several weeks, her skin was healed. With this phase of care complete, the formula was further modified to coordinate with Tamoxifen, the antiestrogen hormonal therapy. The herbs that strongly clear excess, toxic heat were removed as the potential injury from radiation was no longer a risk. *Liu wei di huang wan* continued as the foundation,

---

[131] Jia *et al.*, 2013
[132] Lahans, 2007

Liu Wei Di Huang Wan (Six Ingredient Pill) 60 g	nourish *yin*, reduce estrogen
zhe bei mu (fritillaria thunbergii) 8 g	phlegm-resolving
ji xue teng (spatholobus suberectus) 10 g	nourish blood, maintain blood levels
jin ying zi (rosa laevigata fruits) 15 g	astringes, stabilize and consolidate Kidneys
wu wei zi (schisandra) 15 g	astringes, consolidates *Chong* and *Ren*, calms spirit, nourishes Kidneys
gua lou shi (trichosanthes fruit) 8 g	transforms phlegm
pu gong ying (taraxacum mongolicum) 15 g	clear heat toxin, eliminates irradiation
ling zhi (ganoderma) 15 g	nourish heart, calm spirit, facilitates mechanism of radiation[133]
mai men dong (ophiopogon) 12 g	nourish *yin*
zhi mu (anemarrhena) 12 g	nourish *yin*, clear deficient heat
mu li (ostrea shell), *long gu* (fossilised bone) 8 g	descend *yang*

and herbs to benefit blood, *yin*, and spirit were added. Most women adjust to Tamoxifen within 3–6 months, but symptoms fluctuate as the hormonal integrity resets in the system. Therefore, ongoing modifications should be expected to support the transition.

The Clinical Challenges

A core pillar of the IO paradigm is collaboration among disciplines. This is difficult to achieve when clinicians are spread out among sites, not connected by institutions or established networks. Patients often become the messengers, moving between providers and sharing information with their integrative team in an attempt to coordinate care. Thus, while seamless communication is an ultimate goal, its practical application has yet to be realized. In an oncology-focused practice, we are committed to establishing connections with our conventional medicine colleagues to discuss shared patient treatment goals. This becomes even more important with herbal medicine, because it is the TCM modality that raises the most concern. As part of the patient's initial intake, collect the treating oncologist's practice information as well as other healthcare providers.

---

[133] Lahaus, 2007

With herbal integration, create a document that outlines botanical ingredients and purpose of herbs during conventional treatment for the oncologist. Research singular herbs, reference and cite studies that provide scientific basis when available. For example, we have used the herb database provided by the integrative medicine department at Memorial Sloan Kettering Cancer Center for oncologists. Hundreds of botanicals are listed by common name and indicate function, mechanism of action and potential herb-drug interactions. Write a professional letter of introduction to the oncologist or medical provider. Include information about your clinical practice, experience in TCM oncology and herbal medicine for cancer, and provide medical reasoning as to why the patient would benefit from Chinese herbs during conventional treatment. Suggest an opportunity to speak in more detail.

In several instances, we have provided a list of recommended herbs or formulas to oncologists for review and approval. We include the TCM function and translate these terms into an accessible medical language. The addition of scientific references or studies is also an opportunity to highlight the botanical properties and demonstrate how they have been analyzed. In cases where the herbal prescription is cycled in conjunction with the allopathic treatments, indicate the timing and the clinical reasoning. If there are known side-effects to a particular chemotherapy which a single herb will mitigate, describe the benefits.

Patient compliance is another challenge in herbal integrative oncology. And yet, there is no greater reward for TCM doctors than when patients take their herbs. We recognize the therapeutic value of herbal medicine, but it's inherently difficult invoking that same enthusiasm into patients. This is even more difficult to navigate in cancer management. Patient compliance is a moving target for a variety of reasons. In the course of learning how to best integrate formulas into treatment plans, we continued to come up against specific obstacles that occurred *after* a prescription was filled. We assumed patients made an informed decision to integrate herbs. All questions had been answered. They were prepared to follow the dosing guidelines mapped out in conjunction with conventional protocols. Despite this, we found some patients were not taking their herbs as prescribed or at all.

Often, this relates to taste and ease of ingestion. There are several forms of herbal prescription: raw, granulated powders and encapsulated or pill form. The "taste complaint" does not factor in with the pills or encapsulated herbs. The metabolic intake of herbs in pill form is slower and more cumulative. As a result, we prefer granular powders or raw herb form because of greater therapeutic potency. This also allows for cyclical dosing and herbal modification. There are two aspects that tend to inhibit compliance. First, some individuals have highly sensitive palates who cannot seem to tolerate the taste of powdered herbs. It is not uncommon to hear colorful commentary on the flavor profile of the herb formula. Some of our favorites, "It's like moldy dish water," or "It reminds me of horse manure and nail polish." The descriptions are quite entertaining. There is either an attempt for a period of time to acclimate to the taste, or they quit and ask for another option.

At that point, we revert to encapsulated granules. The challenge with this form of tailored formulas is dosing. Generally, 500 mg fill one capsule. In order to take a therapeutic dose, handfuls of capsules are required. For example, a patient diagnosed with pancreatic cancer was prescribed an herbal formula but was extremely sensitive to the taste. The aversion was so intense, she continued to miss her doses. As a compromise, she insisted on encapsulated herbs. But, it required her to take 23 per day. This is not easily achieved particularly when digestion is impaired and the Spleen and Stomach is weak. In the end, she did not take herbs.

Cytotoxic therapy frequently causes nausea and vomiting. Acute symptoms are largely controlled by anti-nausea medications. Despite this, an underlying current of digestive sensitivity inhibits desire to eat, which leads to weight loss, something that must be monitored in active treatment. Constant, low-grade nausea corresponds to Stomach *yin* deficiency and Spleen/Stomach deficiency patterns. When this occurs, even sweet tonics to support the Spleen and Stomach to regulate digestion and tonify deficiency, trigger stomach upset. If a patient happens to take herbs and vomits, all bets are off. This is when it is profoundly useful to research the expected side-effects of cytotoxic medicine to pre-emptively support digestion (Spleen *qi* and Stomach *yin*) and counteract acute physical responses.

"I've completed chemotherapy. Do I need to keep taking herbs?" Unequivocally, the answer is always "yes." In our clinical expertise, the most significant phase of treatment occurs when the Western treatment plan is complete. It is a window of opportunity to optimize recovery separate from the presence of disease or its interventions. Understandably, patients have also their limit of medical interventions. Even a sensitivity to acupuncture is heightened, as one patient commented, "I don't think I can take any more poking. I know this is good for me, but after so many different treatments at the hospital, I need a break." While we like to consider that TCM is gentle and supportive, it is still a therapeutic modality. For those who have endured months, sometimes years of ongoing cancer treatment, there is a point when a desire to scale back interventions even those that are holistic.

The value of practicing a system of medicine with multiple healing modalities is the versatility. When we are asked if continuing herbs is necessary, we clarify the role of herbal medicine specific to their health. Even if there is no indication of cancer, it is important to support the healing process in order to establish a healthy physiological terrain. We explain how the recovery phase is as important as the treatment phase because the body is rebuilding for months and years after cancer treatment. Further, herbs are a form of preventative medicine. By strengthening and harmonizing vital substances in the body, disease struggles to manifest. The same type of conversation is applicable when asked if herbs are necessary to continue in between chemotherapy cycles before or after surgery. Our experience shows that patients want to understand and are very much involved in their healthcare decision-making process.

A secondary component to herbal medicine correlates to an unfortunate reality that plants are for profit. We can only blame pharmaceutical companies for so much because there are many herb manufacturers who are in the business to make money as well. Across the board, herbs are exponentially more cost effective than any aspect of cancer treatment, but herbs are not capable of curing cancer in its entirety. The expense of conventional medicine treatments is costly, and this causes financial strain on many families. This awareness is embedded in the psychosocial concepts of IO, which considers the high costs associated with treatment of the disease. Complementary and alternative medicine modalities can exploit the patient, promising curable outcomes at high costs. This is another reason the IO community created a formidable definition and guidelines for patients to rely on safe practices, and practitioners to follow.

The cost of herbal medicine trickles down to the Chinese medicine doctor's pharmacy. The decision to upcharge from wholesale herbal costs is common practice though there are varying degrees of the profit margin. There is also an evident trend in an increase in herb prices throughout the industry. This has an indirect effect on the consumer, who is also the cancer patient. On many occasions, patients who are on tight budgets will be able to take herbs (at cost) for a certain period of time, but then not refill their order because of limited funds. This makes herbal prescription prohibitive for many. Providers must remain aware of the psycho-social components in patient care, and when possible, make accommodations to improve accessibility. There is no outright solution to this problem, but it is a crucial consideration for Chinese herbalists committed to the incorporation of plant medicine for the management of cancer.

Chinese herbal medicine is innately whole. The pharmacopeia established thousands of years ago by wise sages and herbalists in China is a highly valuable modality and resource in the treatment of modern diseases. Its ability to complement conventional treatments to strengthen the body's terrain throughout phases of cancer is unsurpassable. It is inherently based in empirical research and within that, Science. Its efficacy is evident by way of clinical technique and refinement. This chapter has attempted to offer a practical framework for application, methods the TCM practitioner can employ to formulate an herbal prescription that aligns with the physiological presentation. For a more in-depth examination and application of Chinese herbs and cancer, we highly recommend the advanced clinical text written by Dr. Tai Lahans, L.Ac. entitled, *Integrating Conventional Chinese Medicine in Cancer Care: A Clinical Guide*. It is an exceptional contribution to the art and science of herbs for cancer management. The versatility of plant medicine must be recognized, as herbs are integral components in the synergistic system that is traditional Chinese medicine.

References

Bryan, J. (2011). How bark from the Pacific yew tree improved the treatment of breast cancer. *The Pharmaceutical Journal*. Retrieved September 27, 2018, from https://www.pharmaceutical-journal.com/news-and-analysis/news/how-bark-from-the-pacific-yew-tree-improved-the-treatment-of-breast-cancer/11084729.article?firstPass=false

Chen, J., Chen, T., & Crampton, L. (2004). *Chinese Medicine Herbology and Pharmacology.* City of Industry: Art of Medicine Press.

Chiou, C., Wang, K.C., *et al.* (2018). Liu Jun Zi Tang — A Potential, Multi-Herbal Complementary Therapy for Chemotherapy-Induced Neurotoxicity. *International Journal of Molecular Sciences, 19*(4), 1258.

Cohen. (2015). [Telephone interview].

Gagnier J. J., Boon H., Rochon P., Moher D., Barnes J., & Bombardier C. (2006). Reporting randomized, controlled trials of herbal interventions: An elaborated CONSORT statement. Ann Intern Med. 2006b; 144(5), 364–367. [PubMed] [Reference list]

Jia, L., Ma, S., Hou, X., Qased, A.B., Sun, X., & Fan, F. (2013). The synergistic effects of traditional Chinese herbs and radiotherapy for cancer treatment. *Oncology Letters, 5*(5), 1439–1447. doi:10.3892/Ol.2013.1245.

Lahans, T. (2007). *Integrating Conventional and Chinese Medicine in Cancer Care: A Clinical Guide.* Philadelphia, PA: Churchill Livingston Elsevier.

McCulloch, M., & See C. (2006). Astragalus-based Chinese herbs and platinum-based chemotherapy for advanced non-small cell lung cancer: Meta-analysis of randomized trials.

Morelle, R. (2016). Kew Report Makes New Tally for Number of World's Plants. Retrieved September 7, 2018, from https://www.bbc.com/news/science-environment-36230858

Newman, D. J., Cragg, G. M., & Snader, K. M. (2003). Natural Products as Sources of New Drugs over the Period 1981–2002. *Journal of Natural Products, 66*(7), 1022–1037. doi:10.1021/np030096l

Peiwen, L. (2003). *Management of Cancer with Chinese Medicine.* St. Albans, Herts, UK: Donica Publishing Ltd.

Qu, Z., Cui, J., Aung, T., *et al.* (2016). Identification of Candidate Anti-Cancer Molecular Mechanisms of Compound Kushen Injection Using Functional Genomics. *Oncotarget.* doi: https://doi.org/10.18632/oncotarget.11788

Rashrash, M., Schommer, J. C., & Brown, L. M. (2017). Prevalence and Predictors of Herbal Medicine Use Among Adults in the United States. *Journal of Patient Experience, 4*(3), 108–113. https://doi.org/10.1177/2374373517706612

Rugo, H., Shtivelman, E., Perez, A., Vogel, C., Franco, S., Tan Chiu, E., *et al.* (2006). *Phase I trial and antitumor effects of BZL101 for patients with advanced breast cancer.* Spring Science +Business.

Schiff, P. B., & Horwitz, S. B. (1980). Taxol stabilizes microtubules in mouse fibroblast cells. *Proceedings of the National Academy of Sciences USA, 77*(3), 1561–1565. doi: https://doi.org/10.1073/pnas.77.3.1561

Tianqi W., Xianjun F., & Zhenguo W. "Danshen Formulae for Cancer: A Systematic Review and Meta-Analysis of High-Quality Randomized Controlled Trials," Evidence-Based Complementary and Alternative Medicine, vol. 2019, Article ID 2310639, 16 pages, 2019. https://doi.org/10.1155/2019/2310639.

University of Adelaide. (2016). How Chinese medicine kills cancer cells. Science-Daily. Retrieved August 30, 2018. Retrieved from https://www.sciencedaily.com/releases/2016/09/160908084319.htm

Wong, B. Y., Lau, B. H., Jia, T. Y., & Wan, C. P. (1996). Oldenlandia diffusa and Scutellaria barbata Augment Macrophage Oxidative Burst and Inhibit Tumor Growth. Cancer Biotherapy and Radiopharmaceuticals, 11(1), 51–56. doi:10.1089/cbr.1996.11.51

Zhu, J., Halpern, G. M., & Jones, K. (1998). The Scientific Rediscovery of a Precious Ancient Chinese Herbal Regimen: Cordyceps sinensis Part II. The Journal of Alternative and Complementary Medicine, 4(4), 429–457. doi:10.1089/acm.1998.4.429

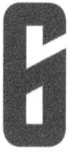

6 Manual Therapy

"It is believed by experienced doctors that the heat which oozes out of the hand, on being applied to the sick, is highly salutary... Thus it is known to some of the learned that health my be implanted in the sick by certain gestures, and by contact, as some disease may be communicated from one to another."

Hippocrates

Manual therapies encompass a range of manipulations traditionally directed towards correcting physical issues, such as posture and alignment, alleviating stagnation or pain, and also to enhance feelings of well-being. Medical massage such as *Tui Na*, partner-assisted stretches, and range of motion (ROM) exercises are all used to open the joints, loosen the muscles and promote circulation both physically and energetically. When used in concert with TCM modalities, such as acupuncture and moxibustion, therapeutic change is often quickly achieved. Patients report a decrease in pain, and physical mobility along with feelings of well-being are enhanced.

In our clinics, we typically use a combination of massage, stretching and range of motion exercises with our cancer patients who complain of muscle stiffness, tightening of tissue (often associated with radiation exposure), neuropathy and stress-related tension. In general, the therapeutic application of these methods is divided into two categories according to the phase of cancer:

- Active phase: chemotherapy or radiation cycles
- Recovery phase: time period from completion of treatment up to one year

Active Phase

During active chemotherapy or radiation treatment, it is advisable to avoid manual techniques which are intense, such as the Graston Technique in physical therapy or deep tissue massage. These methods utilize a significant amount of pressure that can further inflame or damage an area of injury. For example, skin that is red or peeling from radiation should not be manipulated with manual techniques. In addition, the physical side-effects of cytotoxic therapies lower blood chemistry values, such as white or red blood cells. This systemic response indicates heightened susceptibility of musculoskeletal sensitivity and a tendency toward soreness and bruising. Thus, vigorous styles of bodywork are contraindicated. The cumulative depletion that occurs as a result of cyclical therapies causes a wide range of weakness as well. While some individuals with strong constitutions maintain moderate energy levels and stamina through treatment, others suffer greatly and find it difficult to simply get out of bed. For the latter, these patients are at higher risk of fainting with any type of vigorous modality, whether acupuncture or manual therapy techniques.

We have found less is more and focus on gentle stretching with passive range of motion techniques, or gentle therapeutic massage methods. These are performed in order to maintain healthy circulation, relax the patient and impart feelings of well-being. Therapeutic touch is nurturing and soothing, and for a cancer patient, these are crucial elements to healing since so much of their experience is shrouded in invasive, often painful, treatments. However, manual therapy does more than just promote "feel-good" responses. Specific approaches establish healthy circulatory functions that offset the tendency of the body's structure to tighten up, spasm or overprotect a compromised area. Acute lumbar pain, fibrotic tissue or neuropathy can all be addressed with careful manipulation. Patients' pain levels will decrease, and they may feel more relaxed.

Recovery Phase

In the recovery phase, massage tends to take a more prominent place in this aspect of manual therapy techniques. The level of massage is dictated by the relative strength and sensitivity of the patient. The further away from chemotherapy or radiation, the stronger the body becomes, but the recovery phase can last years, depending on the diagnosis and extent of total treatments. A complete assessment of the whole person considers the Chinese medical diagnoses in accordance with physical presentations. For example, in cancers of the breast, the patient may experience shoulder or arm discomfort related to side-effects of radiation. A common presentation is cording or fibrosis that leads to involuntary guarding of the affected area and ranges of immobility. Left untreated, or ignored, the healthy tissue becomes further compromised and tightening, inflammation and pain persist. The platinum-based chemotherapeutic agents induce neuropathy in the hands and feet, which can present within weeks of infusions and continue years past treatment. The location of a tumor and potential metastatic spread is another indicator of possible pain patterns.

It behooves the practitioner to become familiar with the conventional treatments and potential side effects to strengthen the body in a preventative manner and to lessen the degree to which symptoms occur. Equally important is recognizing the onset and earliest signs of imbalance. When a patient says they do not have signs of neuropathy, but then casually refer to the slight numbness at the tip of their fingers, this is a clear sign that neuropathic side-effects are surfacing and must be addressed. The earlier a practitioner is aware of the manifestation of symptoms before they cause an inordinate amount of problems and pain, the more advantageous for the patient's healing process. This approach reflects the therapeutic value of collaborative care and enhances the role of Chinese medicine within integrative oncology methods. The following section outlines three fundamental practices that are used effectively.

Massage

There are innumerous treatment cautions in cancer management designed to protect the patient from practices that are potentially harmful. Massage was not an exception to this debate. Concerns whether bodywork caused spread of cancer cells were voiced, but there is simply no credible evidence to this theory. That being said, aggressive or inappropriately applied massage techniques have the capacity to induce local inflammation, soreness or even bruising. This technique paired with a weak, deficient patient will lead to further depletion, which is not an ideal outcome. Therefore, the following outlines basic cautions and considerations for safe, therapeutic application:

- Positioning of the patient: Be cognizant of the positioning of the patient with respect to surgeries and/or skin sensitivities (e.g. radiation) from treatment.
- Strength of the techniques: Keep in mind that the patient may be more physically sensitive and in a weakened state.
- Lymphedema: There are specific techniques that should be used for lymphedema as traditional massage techniques may make it worse.
- Do not massage a tumor directly or over the site of a tumor: There is no definitive evidence that the cancer cells will spread, but it will likely be physically and emotionally uncomfortable for the patient.

Tui Na

In TCM, historically, *Tui Na* has been used as the primary manual therapy alone and/or in conjunction with other modalities to treat conditions such as orthopedic disorders, pediatric complaints, and internal and gyneco-logical illnesses. The techniques of *Tui Na* are based on the principles of TCM and work by regulating *yin* and *yang*, *qi* and blood to reinforce deficiencies and reduce excess to rectify physical abnormality. The *Tui Na* that people experience in the West is often very different than an experience in China. For one, our laws are different. The *Tui Na* practitioner in China, for example, would traditionally include bone setting as part of their repertoire. Also, their techniques are more aggressive. In the United States, manipulation of bones is strictly contraindicated by anyone other than licensed chiropractors, doctors of osteopathy, etc.

While there are many techniques that encompass the system of *Tui Na*, some of the more common modes include: Pressing (*an fa*), Kneading (*rou fa*), Friction (*mo ca fa*), Flicking and Plucking (*tan bo fa*), and Traction and Rotation (*qian yin fa* and *yao fa*). Pressing is a movement typically done with the belly of the thumb or palm, but the tip of the middle finger can also be used. Most often it is used to target specific acupressure points, *ashi* points, or areas of tightness. Kneading utilizes the whole palm or elbow/forearm; however, the thumb or two-thumb combination can also be used. This technique strongly invigorates *qi* and blood or subdues *yang* depending on the location and intensity of the technique. Friction is typically applied with the palm to address cold conditions, to release the exterior, or move *qi* in a channel. Flicking and plucking uses the fingers on long and hard tissues or muscles. Traction and rotation treat impaired mobility of joints as well as muscle and tissue tension.

Stretching

From the sarcomeres to the connective tissue to the realignment of disorganized fibers, the science behind stretching is actually quite interesting. However, most people are not interested in *how* a muscle stretches but in *how to* stretch. Stretching is often associated with exercise, an activity done to warm-up muscles and cool down after exertion. As such, over the years many stretching methods have been developed and typically fall into one of two categories:

- Static: the person stretches with no movement
- Dynamic: the person stretches with movement. In this section, we are not concerned with methods that optimize athletic improvement. Instead, it focuses on stretching approaches that allow the musculature of the body to release and lengthen with the goal of improving movement, circulating *qi* and blood and reducing pain.

In general practice, when a patient complains of pain or tightness, we ask if they stretch. The answer is not a resounding "yes, all the time!" A majority of patients have completed a series of physical therapy sessions at some point for acute or chronic injury, which has laid a foundation of the function and purpose of stretching. However, despite varying degrees of discomfort and limited ROM, daily stretching practices are hard to come by. Despite this reality, stretching is crucial in the restoration and health of the body, so we inquire about the type and the frequency they stretch. It is also quite helpful to say, "show me how you stretch." The most common method is the random, quick, cold stretch when a person feels tight or has a body ache. Some claim they stretch all of the time, and many respond to the question of stretching with, "I do yoga." With this response, we gently remind the patient that while there are many benefits of a regular yoga practice, it has changed over the years, and some disciplines focus on strengthening above stretching. It is important to clarify the style of yoga they practice in order to determine the degree of stretching involved. Yoga is not always a substitute for simple stretching, though it is a practice we encourage to regulate *qi* and calm the mind.

There are many stretching variations dependent on the orthopedic condition and patient health. While we provide basic stretching exercises for self-care, we put more emphasis on *how* to stretch, and its unique effect when done correctly. In clinic, we demonstrate and incorporate static and dynamic stretching exercises. Typically, the dynamic aspect is a self-care tool that can be practiced regularly throughout the day and in conjunction with physical exercise routines. Static stretching methods are extremely useful in clinic, and a modality that enables the practitioner to provide therapeutic release. It is particularly effective when a patient is too sensitive for needles but can withstand gentle movement and mild treatment. Depending on the goals and flexibility of the patient, we will typically begin with the basic technique of stretch and hold, and then progress to passive (assisted) stretching, active stretching and various types of isometric stretching.

The differences between standard stretching protocols and more advanced isometric exercise relate to movement. With the former, a person can flow from one stretch to another after holding it for a predetermined amount of time, or even repeat the stretch if more attention is needed in a particular area. This process can be achieved daily to lengthen and relax the body. By contrast, isometric stretching is passive and involves the contracting and stretching of specific muscles. To execute an isometric release, the muscle is contracted for approximately 15 seconds before it is released and stretched again. This delivers a relatively deeper stretch than previously allowed, where it is held for another 20–30 seconds.

The contraction phase is enhanced with a person or object resisting the contraction and any movement. This entire process is typically repeated anywhere from 2–5 times. Compared to basic static hold stretching, this technique can provide the added benefits of increasing range of motion and building strength through the micro-contractions within the muscle itself. Therefore, it is a good form of conditioning for cancer patients who want to exercise but have been limited due to their illness. With this in mind, we recommend this type of stretching no more than three days per week to allow the body to rest and recover between each session.

Just as TCM looks at each person individually, the same approach needs to be taken with stretching. It is necessary to consider the cofactors that influence the ability to stretch, including:

- medical conditions
- level of fitness
- prior injuries
- scar tissue
- muscle fatigue
- level of hydration or dehydration
- various age-related issues such as elastic or collagen content, etc.

Cancer-specific concerns relate to active chemotherapy or radiation cycles, location of disease, metastatic spread, medications, concurrent cancer-related issues and energy levels. Tracking this health information is an integral component to formulating the proper stretching exercise as an effective complementary modality. Based on the patient's diagnosis and presenting symptoms, the practitioner can incorporate these methods in clinic and as home-care. Consistency, duration and breathing are key aspects to healthy stretching that are important to review with patients, which are outlined below.

Consistency

Stretching is an empowering tool that enhances the body's ability to adapt and change over a period of time. The results of stretching unfold in a systematic manner, allowing the physical structure of the body to catalogue its benefits and then more easily respond. Consistency is key, so results are noticeable and achieved through lighter, but more frequent routines. Essentially, there is more long-term benefit derived from stretching regularly for 5–10 minutes a day, compared to a more intense one hour stretching session a week. In cancer management, we prescribe mild stretching, several times a week depending on the phase of treatment. During the recovery phase, it is an optimal time to reintroduce exercise and stretching slowly and cumulatively as the body repairs and rebuilds.

Duration

There are varying opinions on how long a stretch should be held. On average, the recommended range is 30 seconds to over two minutes. Regardless, we observe that most patients are not holding their stretches nearly long enough. Most tend to release as soon as there is an element of discomfort, which somehow signals that the result has been achieved, and this release is too soon. This does not facilitate much lasting change in the muscle and its attachments. We start with encouraging at least 30 seconds and up to a minute or more, depending on diagnosis, health and goals. With age, a longer duration often yields greater benefit over time to offset stiff, tight muscles. The sensation that accompanies a longer hold and proper stretch can vary, but feelings of warmth and a relative lengthening of muscle ensue.

Breathing

One of the most common occurrences with stretching is a tendency to hold the breath. Muscles need oxygen to repair and release. So, holding of the breath impairs this restorative function. Slower, deep breathing is optimal. We have our patients count out loud while stretching because it forces a more natural respiration and cycle of breath. The counting also forces accountability in holding the stretch for the appropriate amount of time.

Cautions and Recommendations

Stretching is a form of exercise. Therefore, the same precautions and recommendations one takes when starting a new exercise routine should be taken with stretching. Precautions such as:

- Warm up properly — Depending on the routine this can be five minutes of walking, easy range of motion exercises, etc.
- Take it slow and ease into the routine — Although 30 seconds is a general goal for stretching, and eventually longer holds are necessary, it is important to learn the alignment, find the breath, and slowly stretch. This is crucial for patients in acute active cancer treatment with relative weakness. Breaking up the sets also gains better ability to safely hold

the stretch longer, such as three sets of 10 second holds. Patients with limited range of motion have progressed from only being able to stretch for a few seconds, to eventually regaining full range of motion and easily holding the stretch for over a minute. This reinforces the concept of consistency.

- Soreness is a potential side-effect of stretching — If it is overdone, just like with other forms of exercise, stretching can cause microscopic damage to the muscle fibers and soreness can occur. Staying well hydrated eases the elasticity of the body and heat applications on the local area for 20–30 minutes will increase the blood flow, which helps flush out chemical irritants contributing to the pain, as well as bringing oxygen and healing nutrients to the location.[134] Local heat application is not advised over tumors and radiation burns.

Sotai

Sotai is a form of movement therapy intended to align the body and correct structural imbalances. It was developed by the late Keizo Hashimoto, M.D., from Japan. It utilizes various exercises and stretches to break holding patterns and re-educate the nervous and muscular systems. Dr. Hashimoto was one of the early pioneers who integrated Oriental medicine's knowledge and philosophy of healing and the body with Western medicine's knowledge and understanding of its functions. A unique example of integrative medicine, he connected TCM's theoretical principles of opposites, *yin-yang* theory and its acumen on the physical body to Western medicine's anatomical and physiological understanding.

Sotai stretching is an example of reciprocal inhibition, the concept of oppositional movement. When the prime muscle (agonist) contracts, the muscles in opposition to it (antagonist) relax and lengthen. For example, the quadriceps comprise four muscle groups in the upper thigh. They tend toward being very tight from physical activity, exertion and walking. The antagonist to the quadriceps is the hamstrings. When the quadriceps contracts to extend the knee then the hamstring needs to relax and lengthen to allow the movement. The opposite is true for knee flexion. The hamstrings,

---

[134] Sarnataro, 2003

as well as the calf, engage and as the knee bends, the quadriceps relax to allow the movement to occur. Engaging the hamstrings and calf so that the quadriceps is in a state of lengthened relaxation, especially with resistance, for a few seconds and then focusing on total body relaxation can help to relax the tight quadriceps.

Sotai is well-suited for the cancer patient because its therapeutic range encompasses qualities that make it an efficient form of stretching, easy to learn and increases comfort. The basic premise is that a person should move in the direction that is comfortable (i.e., does not cause pain). For example, in cases of back pain, if laying down and twisting left causes pain, but twisting right does not, then the stretch will take place on the right side. By going in the comfortable direction, utilizing an isometric contraction followed by a rapid and complete relaxation with exhalation of the breath, then alignment and normalization can return. If executed properly, the patient should notice a significant, if not total, reduction in pain, improvement in alignment, such as leg length for example, and an increase in range of motion. The isometric contraction should take place for approximately a slow three count. At times this process needs to be repeated a few times for optimal effectiveness. Dr. Hashimoto says the secret to sotai is to comfortably and easily move the body to the point where comfort ends, hold for a few seconds, and then rapidly relax and release all force.[135]

Interestingly, a fundamental aspect to this method corresponds to internal relaxation to optimize the external response. If the patient does not release into the stretch, then the result is lessened. If this occurs, we focus on the end of the three count, cue a deep inhale, and then exhale completely as they rapidly relax the entire body. The role of the practitioner is to give resistance in the isometric contraction phase. This forces the muscles to contract, perhaps even fatigue, and it is then guided to facilitate a complete release.

Synergistic Treatments

Fortunately, there are a myriad of manual therapy techniques available to the practitioner in clinical practice. When used in conjunction with TCM modalities, such as acupuncture, outcomes are further enhanced and often

---

[135] Hashimoto, 1981

occur with minimal focused effort. However, treatments for cancer-related conditions require close examination and attention. The TCM physician must be familiar with the Western diagnosis, treatment plan and patient's response to such treatments. Consider the integrated diagnosis to bridge the gap among modalities and formulate a balanced plan. For instance, when a patient is too sensitive for even a gentle Japanese-style acupuncture treatment, yet also has significant physical obstacles, the practitioner must devise an approach that increases stamina or *qi*, to enable the body to receive treatment and resolve pain. In cases such as these, gentle range of motion techniques in combination with moxibustion is a complete treatment that promotes circulation and nourishes. For severe cases of neuropathy, acute pain or paralysis, Scalp acupuncture methods with manual therapy is very effective. This approach relies upon refined needle stimulation that influences a central nervous system response with active movements or during manual therapy techniques.

Radiation fibrosis is a recalcitrant condition as a result of radiation therapy. It can occur months after a patient's radiation treatments and continue to progress for years after. The tissue becomes significantly tight, dense and immobile and develops in regions of the body exposed to external beam radiation therapy. It causes the formation of reactive oxygen species (ROS) and direct DNA damage.[136] A combination of manual therapy techniques with moxibustion, pricking therapy, and concurrent use of Master Tung points, such as 77.05, 77.06 and 77.07 for axillary/chest cording can hasten the recovery from this painful condition and act as a matter of prevention.

TCM Integration with Physical Therapy

There is a powerful synergistic quality between the practice of physical therapy (PT) and TCM. Likely because PT is a science-based practice with proven measurements, it is readily accepted and recommended by medical doctors. Of the cancer patients we have worked with, many have been referred to a physical therapist already. This suggests that those patients have received daily exercises and stretches appropriate to their condition.

---

[136] Straub et al., 2015

In these cases, we encourage the patient to continue following the recommendations of the PT and align our approach accordingly. This integration enhances patient mobility, comfort and improves outcomes.

That being said, how does this integration occur? There are a variety of ways to collaborate and blend PT into a Chinese medicine treatment regimen. The deciding factor is often the patient, who recognizes how their body responds to both disciplines. Some prefer to spread out the PT and TCM appointments on different days. This happens mainly with weak patients in active phases of cancer treatment. In such cases, we advise scheduling TCM treatment *before* PT in order to tonify *qi* and also relax the body before more active therapy. By contrast, TCM can be very effective in reducing inflammation, preventing soreness and integrating the work from a PT session.

In conclusion, methods of manual therapy are frequently cautioned in patients with cancer, but the licensed TCM physician has the scope and ability to provide safe, therapeutic treatments as adjunctive therapy. There are many benefits the patient can derive from massage techniques, stretching and *Sotai* exercises, especially in combination with TCM modalities that potentiate the effects of another. Massage and stretching are ways to move the *qi* and blood of the body to help reduce pain without overly taxing or contributing to the fatigue of the patient. This pillar is integral to the physiological terrain of the body and deeply empowers the patient to focus inward to connect with the structural self and promote healing and recovery.

References

Hashimoto, K. (1981). *Sotai, Natural Exercise*. Chico, CA: George Ohsawa Macrobiotic Foundation.

Russi Sarnataro, B. (2003). Sore Muscles? Don't Stop Exercising. Retrieved September 26, 2018, from https://www.webmd.com/fitness-exercise/features/sore-muscles-dont-stop-exercising#3

Straub, J. M., New, J., Hamilton, C. D., Lominska, C., Shnayder, Y., & Thomas, S. M. (2015). Radiation-induced fibrosis: Mechanisms and implications for therapy. *Journal of Cancer Research and Clinical Oncology, 141*(11), 1985–1994. doi:10.1007/s00432-015-1974-6

7 Chinese Nutrition and Dietary Therapy

"Those who take medicine and neglect their diet waste the skill of the physician."

Chinese Proverb

Hippocrates, known as the father of modern medicine, famously said, "Let food be thy medicine and medicine be thy food." In TCM, food therapy, as we refer to diet and nutrition, has remained a prominent part of the medicine as reflected in its inclusion as one of the five pillars of traditional Chinese medicine. Some people even speculate that herbology, which is arguably the most historically prominent pillar in TCM, grew out of a natural evolution of using food to maintain health and treat disease. Although modern medicine still recognizes the role of diet in maintaining health, it has in large part removed it as a form of *therapy*, or healing, as referenced by Hippocrates.

Given the importance of both Eastern and Western medical traditions once placed on food and health, one might think that it would be one of the most evolved aspects of medicine today. However, one could easily argue that nothing is further from the truth. There is probably as much confusion around diet and nutrition as ever before. Possibly this is because diet has become its own industry worth more than 70 billion dollars and is largely focused on physical appearance versus core metrics of health.[137] When it comes to diet, nutrition and cancer, there seems to be even more confusion. To begin with, when we ask a patient if they discussed diet and nutrition with their oncologist,

---

[137] Roepe, 2018

it's common to hear only basic recommendations (plant-based, no sugar, etc.) At best, we are occasionally told that the patient was referred to a nutritionist for a consult. Typically, these consults are along the lines of handing the patient a list of food items to help counteract the nutritional deficiencies that patients can encounter with certain chemotherapies. For example, patients tend to have low-levels of potassium as they go through treatment, so it is recommended by nutritionists to eat certain pre-packaged, frozen, processed meals that have high levels of potassium added. Nutritional shakes are commonly approved because of their relatively high-calorie content and infusion of vitamins. These are not foods we would think of for long-term health and certainly not for already debilitated health in fighting a complex disease.

Nutritionists and dieticians provide a significant amount of resources and information in an accessible manner, customized to the patient for various endemic problems. In the West, food is not typically seen as medicinal, though recent trends indicate a broader lens of understanding with dietary intake and health. Chinese medicine assesses the dietary approach of the patient to optimize health according to their constitution and current condition. Looking at categories, properties and even energetic temperature of food and fluids with patients provides further insight into dietary therapy. What we ingest, elicits a biochemical effect through metabolic function. Quite simply, food causes side-effects, whether desirable or not. This might sound strange because we generally associate the term side-effect with pharmaceuticals. But if food is medicine, as Hippocrates suggested early on, then it's not so strange.

Allergic reactions to ingredients is as an extreme example of a side-effect. Inflammation, is a more subtle and often systemic response as a result of eating certain foods, can also be thought of as a side-effect. Referring back to the examples of foods recommended for cancer patients, the irony is these contain food additives and preservatives introduced during the processing stage to add nutrition and to prolong the shelf life. A 2015 study on food additives and mice suggest a link between some additives and inflammation, weight and metabolism.[138] The link between cancer and inflammation can be traced back to 1863, with modern research data supporting the critical factor that inflammation has in tumor progression. More specifically, "It is now becoming clear that the tumor microenvironment,

---

[138] Torgan, 2018

which is largely orchestrated by inflammatory cells, is an indispensable participant in the neoplastic process, fostering proliferation, survival and migration."[139] Our traditional Chinese medicine view of processed foods, as we have experienced it in our clinics, is that processed foods tend to be damp-producing. This dampness is likely produced from either an over-abundance of *yin*/fluid-like ingredients or, more likely, from our body's inability to digest and assimilate the food. When dampness accumulates, it becomes phlegm, a more substantial form of damp and damp-phlegm, which is one diagnostic quality attributed to tumors in TCM.

Putting this together from a modern Western view, we see processed food can cause inflammation in the body, and inflammation is likely a key component to tumor proliferation. In TCM, unchecked dampness evolves into phlegm, causing a cascade of disrupted *qi* and blood flow, leading to greater stagnation of phlegm, *qi* and blood. Ultimately, creating an environment that may encourage tumor formation. This is an oversimplification of the tumor formation process from both Eastern and Western perspectives. But it illustrates how cumulative exposure to varied substances become contributing factors in the development of disease. In cases of chronic diseases such as cancer, it is usually the accumulative negative effects on the body that lead to an environment susceptible to disease. However, the prevention and the healing of disease can also occur by cumulative intake of healthy food and fluids. Food therapy does not lend itself to an overnight cure, but the long-term benefits are evident and can be very powerful.

TCM Food Therapy

Traditional Chinese medicine aims to maintain or bring back balance to the body. The same is true for its philosophy of *food therapy*. In simple terms, a balanced body is a healthy body, free of disease and pain. Food therapy implies the use of food not just in the maintenance of health but as a modality in the treatment and prevention of disease. The approach is more often focused on the patient's current composition of health rather than a particular symptomatic complaint. For example, where Western nutrition might say eat bananas for cramping, in TCM we would look at the

---

[139] Coussens, 2002

patient's diagnosis to determine the underlying reason for the cramping. In TCM diagnostics this could relate to blood deficiency or pathogenic Liver wind, both of which require unique types of foods for treatment. By comparison, bananas are energetically cooling and very moistening, so they may not be good for someone with *yang* deficiency and damp, which often occurs in late-stage cancer patients. In this way, TCM recognizes that food recommendations will vary depending on the constitutional tendencies and current health of the individual. To do this, TCM looks at the properties of food and how each food affects the body. Considerations include the flavor/taste, energetic thermal nature, which can be manipulated depending on preparation and is another consideration, organ network association, influence on the movement of *qi* in the body (up-bearing, down-bearing, falling, and floating), phase association (Wood, Fire, Earth, Metal, Water), function or effect of the food (e.g. nourish *qi* and blood) and season. In this section, we will look at the considerations for dietary therapy, the various aspects of food properties in TCM and provide general recommendations.

Time of the Year

The current season and weather are important factors. For example, healthy people in winter, which is a *yin* time of year, will want to eat more *yang*, warming food, such as meat to balance out the cold of the season. This was perfectly exemplified on a trip to Mongolia when the husband of our hosting family entered the *ger* (a Mongolian yurt), plopped down a hunk of mutton on our plates, which in TCM is energetically warming, and kicked off dinner by simply stating, "We eat to stay warm." Some may argue that eating and feeling warm is part of thermoregulation of the body between eating and metabolism; however practical application here is important. There is a marked difference in how warm one will feel between eating mutton versus eating an avocado, which is also a fatty food but is energetically cool in temperature. Likewise, in summer, a *yang* time, typically more *yin*, cooling foods are eaten. This is akin to the adage of "Eat what is in season."

Taste — TCM distinguishes tastes or flavors of food. These are sweet, sour, bitter, spicy, and salty. Some also teach of a sixth taste, bland. This covers areas the other five flavors do not. Sweet is associated with the TCM organs of the Spleen and Stomach, sour corresponds with the Liver and Gallbladder, bitter with Heart and Small Intestine; spicy with Lungs and Large Intestine, and salty with the Kidneys and Bladder.

Energetic temperature — Foods may be categorized as cold, cool, neutral, warm or hot in nature. This is an oversimplification, but typically the application is fairly straightforward in that cold diseases would be balanced out with warm or hot food and vice versa for warm diseases.

Preparation — In TCM, food and fluids should be consumed at room temperature, preferably warmer. This is because it is easier to digest, meaning it doesn't have to work as hard and requires less energy, and we are able to assimilate the *qi* of the food with more ease. Cold food or drink from the refrigerator hinders this process. Cold can also cause dampness as well as weakening digestion, which also causes dampness to form. Essentially, one is putting out the "digestive fires" of the middle *jiao*. For instance, blueberries tonify the Liver blood and are antioxidant rich. It is better to steam or cook them versus eating them straight out of the cold refrigerator. There is some debate among practitioners, but generally food preparation from cold to more warming is as follows: raw, steamed, boiled, stewed, stir-fried, baked, deep-fried, roasting.

Side effects — Food causes degrees of reactions in the body, both positive and negative. In TCM, while the sweet taste tonifies and alleviates pain, too much creates damp and should be avoided in Kidney diseases. Sour astringes and engenders fluids and *yin*, but too much makes phlegm worse and should be avoided in Spleen diseases. The bitter taste clears heat and damp-heat, but too much injures the Spleen and *yin*. So it should be avoided in Lung diseases. Spicy scatters and is used to expel pathogens, but too much also injures *yin* and should be avoided in Liver disease. Salty softens hardness and has a downward movement, but too much injures fluids and should be avoided in Heart diseases.

Recommendations

Food as medicine can be a very powerful, albeit long-term, approach. The TCM nutrition approach calls for consistent diagnostic evaluation in order to take into consideration all contributing factors, such as time of year and constitution of the patient. This approach to food is wholly different from the way most of our patients in the West, which is a considerable barrier to fully utilizing this approach in clinical practice. Perhaps this is part of the reason that we support patients in order to encourage them to make meaningful, consistent changes to their diet. It is one of the most difficult aspects of implementing care in our clinics.

This modality is exponentially more challenging in cancer management and during active treatment. Digestive sensitivity is a common cancer-related cofactor. Nausea, vomiting, lack of appetite, mouth sores and taste changes impact desire to eat. While there are therapeutic, nutrient-rich foods and traditional recipes to share, they may all but go out the window for lack of compliance. Ultimately, it is better for a patient to eat and avoid malnutrition or cachexia. In TCM, not eating damages a patient's *qi*, which lowers immunity and vitality. One of the most insightful lessons we learned was from an exceptional oncology dietician with decades of experience. As we observed her intake with an 82 year-old woman undergoing chemotherapy for breast cancer, her family complained that all she wanted were bean burritos from Taco Bell. They were appalled and refused to get them for her, but the dietician told them to allow her to eat it all she wanted. Beans had fiber, the tortilla provided carbs, and cheese provided protein. This was better than the alternative of not eating. So, if nothing else can be managed, we will typically stress the following:

- **Congees/soups/stews:** The underlying theme here is to eat foods that are as easy, and potentially nutritious, as possible to digest. We want the patient to make it as easy as possible for his or her body to take the *qi*, or nutrition, from food and assimilate it into their body. Congee consists of 6 cups rice to 1 cup water and cooked for 2–3 hours until it becomes like porridge. Chinese herbs, spices, meat, eggs or fish can be added to enhance the nutritional value and taste.

- **Bone broth:** Bone broth can be found in use cross-culturally around the world for hundreds if not thousands of years. It is a nutritional panacea. The beef bones should be organic, raised grass-fed *and* finished to yield higher amounts of omega-3s in the broth, which fight inflammation. Preparation is also important, adding in an acid, like apple cider vinegar, will help soften the bones to leach out minerals such as calcium and extract glucosamine and chondroitin sulfate from bones and cartilage, aiding in bone and joint health. Bone broth needs to be consumed consistently to garner many of the long-term health benefits. Some athletes, such as Kobe Bryant, give credit to bone broth for hastening recovery from injuries, which shows the potential for immediate impact.[140] Bone broth is recommended by nutritionists to heal the gut, decrease pain and inflammation and improve the health of hair, skin and nails. Bone broth is indispensable and highly encouraged in cancer care.

Western Diet and Nutrition

In the West, we categorize food into groups then further subdivide the groups based on characteristics and nutrient content. Scientific reasoning is applied to approximate the proportion of nutrients to standardize the food ratios. To monitor our diets, a doctor will order complete blood count (CBC), fasting glucose test and check vitamin levels and cholesterol. This approach is mainly for the purpose of maintaining health and keeping a watchful eye on heart disease and diabetes. Much of the diet and nutrition recommendations that we have in the West are centered around cancer prevention. The most common warn consumers about processed and red meat, but include copious servings of fruits and vegetables, maintain high fiber and low sugar low. This complements maintaining a healthy weight and regular exercise routine. Some of the prospective studies and epidemiologic evidence propose some of these suggestions, such as high fiber and the importance of fruits and vegetables could be overstated.[141]

This answer is likely to be different depending on location, region and cultural background. Various regional/climate, socio-political, religious and cultural views are likely to shape what the perception of a "balanced" diet encompasses. For a long time in America, we were told by our medical and dietary experts to reference the food pyramid as to what a balanced diet should look like. However, it turns out that the original food pyramid, which influenced the way so many of us eat and view balanced nutrition was not based on science but more on what we could produce as a nation to meet our basic caloric needs.[142] This approach took a basic survival attitude of what's easiest and cheapest to produce to meet caloric needs, over a more studied approach of how to optimize our diet to maximize

---

[140] Holmes, 2015
[141] Willett, 2000
[142] Tontonoz, 2016

health. As the science of nutrition has developed we now have a slightly different food pyramid and competing food plate representations on what a healthy, balanced diet should include.

Of course, other factors, such as politics, economics, and some other more unsavory reasons have historically come in to shape the American diet. In 2016, documents were uncovered that showed the sugar industry's concerted effort to manipulate research to put the focus away from sucrose and on saturated fats as the main culprit in heart disease.[143] The concern with respect to cancer is not that sugar causes cancer, but that sugar can be linked to obesity, which is becoming increasingly viewed as a significant contributor to diseases, like cancer.

Western Nutrition and Cancer

While we are not experts in Western nutrition, we have spent the last fifteen years observing trends, following research and speaking with patients on the subject. As it pertains to cancer, it is clear that there is no diet proven to prevent cancer at this time. And, it is unlikely that there will be because there are too many factors involved.

Our intention is not to dismiss the research on diet and cancer. On the contrary, it's very important, but it is just *one* important factor. Research has shown that many of us can benefit from whole-food diets. It has also, at this point, all but confirmed the connection between cancer and processed meats (bacon, sausage, etc.) if over consumed. It has also shed light on issues related to cancer such as obesity. More specifically, that it is not so much the fat we intake but the influence of calories and carbohydrates on obesity.

While there is no cure-all or prevent-all cancers diet, some approaches to eating are showing that they may help with certain cancers. For example, a 2016 review and meta-analyses of the Mediterranean diet with no restriction on fat intake found some evidence that the approach may reduce some incidences of breast cancer, however, but not mortality.[144] The review indicates that a healthy diet is established cumulatively and daily, in a preventative approach. This is similar to other conditions such as heart disease, obesity and diabetes.

---

[143] Kearns, 2016
[144] Bloomfield, 2016

Further insights and food for thought comes from a book by David Servan-Schreiber, MD, called *Anti-Cancer: A New Way of Life*. In the book, he references research that analyzed extracts from foods and their effects on specific types of cancer cells, namely: colon, brain, lung, breast, and prostate. What is interesting is that there was some consistency in the extracts of foods that had greater inhibitory effects: garlic, leeks, scallions, brussels sprouts, cabbage, beets, asparagus, and onions. These all have either *qi* and blood moving or draining damp functions in TCM, which as we have noted are two of the predominant TCM patterns associated with cancer. Here are some key factors:

Key Factors
• **Weight Loss:** The issue of weight loss is a significant but often overlooked factor in cancer survival. Multiple studies have identified outcomes in cancer improve with nutritional intervention, which not only can help a patient maintain weight but also stay on their treatment regimen, have better surgical outcomes and improve the patient's quality of life.[145] Therefore, it is not uncommon to hear the recommendation that patients undergoing cancer treatment need more calories and nutrition to fight and recover from cancer. The side-effects that can come with treatment, such as altered taste, decreased appetite, nausea, vomiting, diarrhea, difficulty swallowing, constipation, and that some cancers inhibit absorption of nutrients all lend to patients entering a calorie and nutritional deficit.
• **Malnutrition:** Treatment toxicity, reduced physical functioning, and decreased survival are all associated with malnutrition in cancer patients. The 2017 Prevalence of Malnutrition in Oncology study concluded malnutrition, weight loss and anorexia are common in cancer patients; as well, the study found, upon a patient's first oncology visit, 51% had nutritional impairment, 43% were at risk of malnutrition, and 64% of patients had lost weight in the prior six months.[146]
• **Cachexia:** Cachexia is considered a wasting syndrome that includes weight loss, loss of appetite, as well as muscle loss. It has been estimated that over 20% of cancer patients' deaths are attributable not solely to the cancer but to cachexia, and although the use of anti-neoplastic agents can help treat cancer they also can make cachexia worse.[147]

[145] National Cancer Institute, 2017
[146] Muscaritoli, 2017
[147] Roepe, 2018

We are frequently asked about plant-based diets for cancer. It is surprising to some that because we practice TCM we do not advocate our patients adopt a vegetarian or vegan diet. To begin with, the exclusion of a group of food known to have nutritional value in the correct proportions cannot be considered "balanced," and TCM advocates balance above all else. Second, considering the statistics and the reality we see in our patients with cancer, those who do have a strictly vegetarian or vegan diet, and keep their level of sugar intake in check, suffer much more with issues related to weight loss, strength and vitality.

Practical Integration

Combining the nutritional philosophy of TCM with what Western science has learned about nutrients and the growing or raising of food makes for a potent modality in healing and recovery. Although some cancer patients become very committed to their diet, it is also overwhelming and difficult to manage seamlessly. Exhaustion combined with access to quick and easy food options lends to poor dietary choices. To avoid this, it is very important to gather as much detail as possible from the patient about their eating habits. It can be easy to gloss over the topic and receive vague answers as well. So we also encourage a detailed food journal to review with the patient. Once you have a good sense of their diet and lifestyle, you can offer customized recommendations. There are exceptional books to refer to as well, such as *Chinese Nutrition Therapy*, *Healing with Whole Foods*, and *The Healing Cuisine of China*. All are good resources in order to share recipes and nutritional ideas with patients. Keep in mind that food therapy is relatively safe. However there are certain foods, such as grapefruit, that are known to interact with a number of medications. Be mindful of these outliers when providing nutritional guidance to patients.

As modern-day practitioners of an Eastern classical medical tradition in the West, we can find that we struggle to balance patient compliance with maximizing the medicinal approaches. The unfamiliarity of TCM, cultural differences and familiar pull of Western medicine can create challenges with patient compliance of TCM recommendations. This is especially true of dietary therapy. Unless a patient is fully onboard with embracing the TCM diet therapy approach, we often do not confound the patient with over emphasizing issues such as temperature. We will emphasize taste, cooking methods along with the categories of food because those components are easier to help guide them. In general, the addition of only one or two foods in their meals will give benefit without too much concern about throwing other TCM diagnostic aspects of their health out of balance. Typically, it is easier for patients if you identify things in their diet to take out or heavily modify and provide them with a few specific additions along with the general guidelines for them to consider; at least in the beginning, as they learn and adjust their habits. Purists may disagree, but we find patient compliance higher this way. The two caveats to this are:

- Spices and very concentrated types of foods can have a significant impact on conditions of heat and cold.
- Cases of extreme heat or cold in the patient necessitate the extra cautions.

Cancer patients are contending with a lot of new information and turmoil. Significant dietary changes are often needed and very important but can cause confusion and be overwhelming. TCM professionals know that there is a lot of overlap in food categories, so we try to keep it as simple as possible in our explanations and recommendations. Here are some examples that patients have found useful:

- While changes such as cutting out dairy, sugar or alcohol can have immediate impacts, chronic issues such as rebuilding vitality or working on damp-phlegm accumulations should be looked at retrospectively, about every four weeks, to note progress or changes.
- Stressing about food is not helpful. Diet is very important but one meal will neither save you nor kill you. The stress about that piece of cake at your daughter's birthday will likely do more damage than the cake itself.
- Tastes or flavors in TCM dietary therapy have many attributes. Refer to the table below for helpful points.

Sweet: Nourishes, strengthens and relaxes
Sweet is often craved after a hard day, emotional event or with mental fatigue. Too much of it and synthetic sources can cause dampness. Considered important if *qi* deficiency, especially of Spleen and Stomach, are indicated by the practitioner.

Salty: Helps dissolve congestion and soften hardened areas in the body
Small amounts help tonify the Kidneys. Do not start adding excessive salt to food or cooking.

Bitter: Helps digestion
Can drain damp, prevent damp from forming and clear heat and toxins. Too much can upset the stomach and be mindful if running on the cold side.

Acrid/Spicy: Typically, warming or hot
Moves *qi*. The dispersing action is thought to help prevent or fight off colds in the early stages. Be mindful if on the warm or dry side.

Sour: Typically, foods are cool in nature
Thought to help the emotional "heat" from stress and anger. Astringes fluid and moistening effect. Thus, be mindful if dampness abounds.

- Don't go overboard. Do not start making everything sweet or bitter depending on what is indicated. Start by reducing a major offender to the condition and adding in one or two foods from the category that is desired at each meal. In the example of damp, cut the dairy out and add in almonds and aduki beans. This eliminates damp caused by the dairy and resolves residual damp with intake of almonds and aduki beans. Plus these two ingredients off-set the protein and calcium loss while also adding beneficial fiber.

- It is better to eat then not eat. Remember, almost all forms of healing involve consistent treatment and time for therapeutic effect to grow. Don't delay dietary changes, or any therapeutic approach, but don't be overly guildridden or concerned if you have an off day either.

To help get practitioners started, or for the concerned patient or family member reading, here are some examples of considerations for damp, blood stagnation, and some thoughts on toxic heat.

Preventing Dampness: Foods to Avoid or Significantly Decrease

Cold foods: iced drinks, ice cream	Raw foods: vegetables, fruit
Alcohol	Greasy, heavy or oily food
Dairy, including eggs	Refined carbohydrates (sugar, white flour)
Most grains; especially wheat and starchy carbohydrates. *Exception: Rye (gluten) and amaranth are good for dampness*	Soy: tofu, soymilk

Reduce meat intake

Suggestions to increase red meat generally come if the patient is weak, heading that way, anemic or is not getting enough protein. Our suggestion usually includes to keep it in the diet in small amounts to maintain strength. An exception might be an intestinal tumor or digestive issues in which we would suggest beef bone broth.

In general, bitter tastes are good to help damp conditions. If there are heat signs, a little bit of salty and cool foods can be indicated. If cold signs dominate, some spicy/acrid and warming foods can further help.

Foods to Help Dry Dampness or Transform Phlegm

Papaya*	Aduki bean
Lettuce	Rye (gluten)
Celery	Amaranth
Turnip	Almonds
Asparagus	Pumpkin
Mushrooms	Tea
Mung bean	Dandelion
White pepper	Chamomile
Vinegar (e.g. apple cider vinegar)	

*Fruit and leaves show possible anti-cancer effects[148]

Keep in mind that many foods that move *qi* and or blood are going to be warm in nature.

Foods to Help Disperse Stagnant Blood

Turmeric	Sweet Rice	White pepper
Cinnamon	Scallion	Coriander
Saffron	Eggplant	Ginger
Vinegar	Aduki Bean	Basil
Rosemary	Spearmint	Leek
Chives	Crab	

With blood stagnation, it is also important to move *qi* in order to move blood.

Foods for *Qi* Stagnation	
Onion	Plum
Garlic	Black Pepper (*seasoning*)
Alcohol (*small amount, too much adds excessive heat and dampness*)	Cabbage
Broccoli	Brussel Sprouts
Beets	Chestnut
Hazelnut	Sweet potato (*This is not always included in this category. It may be included at times because it is helpful in digestion and moving things along in the intestines. However, this could be from its moistening properties over true qi moving. Either way, it is so nourishing and has so many antioxidants to help protect cellular DNA damage that it is hard not to include. Caution in damp conditions.*)
Oats	Trout

Foods and Toxic Heat

Toxic heat is one of the more involved diagnostic patterns to treat with food therapy, and one that a patient should get the most guidance on from their practitioner. Toxic heat is thought by some to be the most serious form of heat. It can certainly present symptomatically with both nutritive (*ying*) and blood (*xue*) level heat symptoms. It can be localized or systemic. There can be marked deficiency, excess or both. Therefore, all five tastes may be needed to varying degrees. Foods on the cool side would be indicated as well as cooler cooking methods. If the patient has less damp and strong digestion, they may be able to eat more raw foods. In many cancer patients, dampness is present to some degree so bitter foods to clear heat and dry damp need to be considered. These foods do not need to always be overtly bitter. Broccoli, for example, is cooling, bitter and has a function of diuresis to flush out excess damp. Strong heat can burn *qi*, blood and *yin* and show a false kind of energy. So sweet foods with their *qi* building and moistening effects, and sour foods with their cooling and nourishing fluid attributes could be used. As well, strong heat can harden phlegm, and so salty foods may be useful to help soften. Even acrid/spicy foods can be helpful when appropriately used to open the pores and vent heat when it is at a more superficial level as with radiation for example.

It is important to avoid the warmest types of cooking found in deep-fried and roasted foods. Steaming is considered by some to be a cooling method of eating. It should be used when possible to aid in the digestion while not adding excessive heat as with other methods. Excessively spicy food or excessive amounts of spicy foods should be avoided. Raw foods and iced drinks may feel great to the patient but the use still needs to be cautioned as too much can put out the fire of digestion and lead to other issues such as dampness.

In TCM, general eating and dietary guidelines typically include:

- Relax, avoid tension and be calm while eating. Do not watch television or read emails.
- Chew food thoroughly. Studies on this vary with conclusions from 30 to 50 times for each bite. The takeaway is to chew more than you are probably doing. Properly chewed food helps the break down and metabolizing of food for better nutrient absorption. In TCM, this is akin to supporting the Spleen *qi*.
- Don't eat too much. The target is 70–80% full. Over eating inhibits the Spleen's transform and transport function of nutrients (*qi*) and creates dampness.
- Do not eat too late at night. There is a greater preponderance for creating damp.
- Eat foods in season where you live.
- Avoid anything listed in the "avoid damp" list above. Also, avoid lengthy fasting or fasting too often.

Here we will cover some of the most frequently asked questions from patients:

What Do You Think of Sugar?

While there may be many reasons to avoid sugar, cancer may or may not be one of them. This touches on one of the most hotly debated areas of cancer. There's a lot of conflicting research and theories around sugar, or more specifically, glucose's involvement in cancer. The idea that cancer has an addiction to sugar probably originated from a study by Otto Warburg in the early 20th century. For a time, this was one of the leading understandings of the cause of cancer, but it was replaced in the early 1950s for more of a molecular biology understanding of cancer, which has led to many of the connections we understand today involving DNA and genetics. On the one hand, it makes intuitive sense that a rapidly growing tumor needs the energy that glucose provides to grow. However, there's also the idea that it is very difficult to "starve" cancer because, excluding people with blood-sugar-regulating issues such as diabetes, our bodies are so efficient at keeping our blood sugar in a certain range that it is difficult to truly become deficient.

While there has been a resurgence in Warburg's theories over the past several years, perhaps in part due to the use of PET scans to help reveal where *some* types of cancers are located by finding areas of the body where cells are consuming extra glucose, there may be some validity to it. The current thinking is trending more towards sugar's role in contributing to obesity and inflammation causing cancer over too much sugar or glucose itself. Sugar does raise insulin levels, which in a chronic elevated state signal the fat cells to pick up fat from the blood stream and store it. Sugar also is a sneaky way to add in extra calories in the form of carbohydrates and an excess of calories can lead to weight gain, which over time leads to obesity. Obesity can cause a chronic state of low-level inflammation. Inflammation is one suspected cause of DNA damage that causes cancer. Of course, sugar leads to inflammation itself, when blood sugar increases, the body increases the number of pro-inflammatory cytokines as well as advanced glycation end products (AGEs) that also trigger inflammation.[149]

In TCM, the flavor of sugar, sweet, is related to the Spleen. The Spleen in TCM is related to digestion. When our digestion system is weakened, we crave things that are sweet because in TCM sweet is tonifying or strengthening to the Spleen. Too much sweetness, however, becomes cloying and causes dampness. Dampness, as we have discussed, is one pathology that TCM associates with tumors and cancer. Typically, with our

---

[149] Basta, 2004

cancer patients, we discourage diets that are damp or anything else that impedes the physical or energetic circulation of the body. Also, keep in mind that during the time when TCM was being developed, the sources of sweet being consumed were natural and most likely in the form of honey and fruit. They likely did not consume the quantities or concentrations of sweeteners that we have today.

There also is the issue of artificial sweeteners. A 2018 study found that ten sport supplements and six artificial sweeteners approved by the FDA (advantame, aspartame, acesulfame potassium-k, sucralose, saccharine, neotame) are toxic to digestive gut bacteria.[150] We have observed in our patients that artificial ingredients, whether added for taste or as part of processing, seem to make food more damp in nature. This can manifest a number of ways: as excess mucus production, gaining weight, sinus congestion, loose stools, etc. Of the potential cascade of detrimental effects on health, one of the more concerning is the potential for artificial sweeteners to bring about glucose intolerance, or high blood glucose levels.[151]

The short answer is balance. More specifically, however, we advocate shying away from sugar when possible. Staying away from sugar promotes balance in the diet. Sugar, it seems, is in everything we buy at the store, from the candy, to the salsa. There's a good chance it has sugar in it. Also, by eating sugar, a person is not providing any benefit to their body. Especially if a person is going through standard care treatments for cancer, it is important to minimize the stress on the body and give it the best opportunity to heal and recover as possible. We understand that many, if not most, of our patients going through chemo seem to have a surge in sugar cravings. Of course, we advocate trying to satisfy those cravings with minimal amounts of natural sources such as honey, but ultimately the stress and worry about it may be as bad, if not worse, than the piece of chocolate that was eaten.

What Do You Think of Meat?

When patients ask us about our thoughts on eating meat, they usually are referring to red meat and specifically, beef. They usually don't know

---

[150] Harpaz, 2018
[151] Lardieri, 2018

that TCM classifies the various types of meat differently. Properties such as temperature, taste, and function/effect make certain meat, or other foods, more appropriate at different times and in various quantities. This makes diet very much unique to the individual and their current state of health, which is often fluctuating especially when a disease such as cancer is present. We won't write in too much detail on this because most practitioners are aware of it, and we find it is not practical for most patients to follow on their own.

Referring back to red meat, this is something that has been largely vilified by most of the Western scientific and dietary community with respect to cancer. There is some credence to this as the International Agency for Research on Cancer (IARC) released a report in 2015 that, after reviewing 800 studies, concluded that processed meat (hot dogs, sausage, etc.) is carcinogenic to humans; specifically, to colorectal cancer. Unfortunately, the report did not discriminate between methods of processing meat. It's likely that nitrates and nitrites have much to do with their outcomes, but because they did not differentiate methods, we do not know if this is true or if natural methods of curing meat are significantly safer or not. It also labeled red meat, to include beef, mutton, horse, lamb, goat, veal and pork, as probably carcinogenic despite limited evidence to such and no direct connection as a cause of cancer.[152] As well, the report estimated that *if* the connection with red meat and cancer were true that comparatively there would be four times as many deaths from air pollution as red meat and twelve times as many deaths from alcohol as red meat.[153] Essentially, the report and many of the studies were not well done and leave many unanswered questions. In our minds, there's not enough evidence to ban meat from the diet entirely.

One issue we often find with studies is that they often do not tell you how much is bad or safe to consume. This may be less of an issue from a TCM standpoint because we recognize that individuals are different and will have different requirements and tolerances, so we recognize some natural fluctuation. However, patients typically appreciate some sort of baseline. The World Cancer Research Fund (WCRF), for example, advises

---

[152] Cleveland Clinic Cancer Care Team, 2015
[153] World Health Organization, 2015

up to 18 ounces of cooked red meat per week and little to no processed meat.[154] Red meat does provide many important nutrients such as vitamin B12, iron, zinc, vitamin D and selenium. In traditional Chinese medicine, the amount of beef a person should eat will vary depending on factors that include their state of health and lifestyle among others. Some of the key qualities of beef are it's warm in nature, tonifies blood, and nourishes the Spleen and Stomach. The strength of the Spleen and Stomach is essential in the health and recovery from disease. It is closely related with digestion in Western thought and is how we take nutrients, or *qi*, from what we eat and drink and assimilate it to stay strong (build *qi* and blood), heal and recover from disease.

Blood is important in TCM for our mental and physical health. Blood is the material foundation of *shen*. When the blood is strong, our mind is healthy and sharp, we are emotionally-balanced, and our organs, meridians and tissues are nourished so that we have a full range of sensations and ease of movement. Thus, the state of our blood is strongly correlated with our physical and mental-emotional health and recovery. While we respect the choices our longtime vegan and vegetarian patients make, we cannot deny that we see this patient population struggle the most with recovery from disease and physical injuries and often need more involved treatment. A couple of the ways that blood can be depleted is through excess work, whether physical, mental or emotional as well as through chronic anxiety, worry and overthinking. Standard care treatments for cancer take a huge toll on a patient, and thus blood deficiency is a consistent diagnostic pattern we see in our patients. This makes efforts to nourish the blood through diet and other means imperative during treatment.

In short, we typically do not discourage patients from eating red meat. The intensity and length of care and recovery for cancer patients necessitates, in our view, all the strengthening and nourishing aspects of food available. The idea that additional calories and nutrition are needed by cancer patients to help their body recover is starting to gain more traction.[155] All this being said, there are caveats on our support of beef specifically and red meat in general:

---

154 World Cancer Research Fund, 2018
155 Tontonoz, 2016

- Red meat needs to be organically raised, grass-fed *and* finished. We are starting to understand that beef is not inherently bad to consume, but the way cattle are raised, fed (for instance, away from their natural diet and plumped up with grain) and the addition of hormones and antibiotics given is damaging.

- Excess consumption of red meat occurs in the Western diet. The amount consumed it, often in large portions, inhibits proper digestion. The recommendation by the WCRF seems reasonable if broken up into smaller, three to four-ounce portions throughout the week. Beef, as a reminder, is warm in nature. So if the patient has a lot of heat signs then reducing quantity of beef as part of the diet will promote more balance.

- Preparation is important. While smoking meat and grilling meat with a nice char is delicious, and can occasionally be enjoyed by a healthy adult, it does carry additional carcinogens.

What about Gluten?

We receive a lot of questions about gluten from our patients, especially as it has become somewhat trendy of a topic over the past few years. With respect to cancer, the questions tend to be around cancer risk and risk of recurrence. The only known connection of cancer and gluten is in people with true gluten sensitivity or celiac disease. These are typically intestinal cancers with some evidence coming up pointing to a possible connection with a more rare form of lymphoma. For people who have some sensitivity to gluten, a positive AGA-IgG or AGA-IgA blood test, but not celiac disease because of a negative EMA-IgA test, there is no evidence of a connection with cancer and gluten. To be clear, there is no known connection, but the studies are few and contradictory at this time. Due to the relationship between inflammation and cancer, we caution patients who have a personal or family history of intestinal cancer and refer them to an oncologist for more specific questions and information. A couple other considerations that can arise with the question of gluten:

- Fructose malabsorption: The symptoms can mimic those of celiac disease, non-celiac gluten sensitivity and IBS. This can be a consideration for patients who test negative in celiac and other gluten sensitivities to bring up to their primary care physician.

- Whole grains: With gluten and without, whole grains have fiber and other nutrients that have been seen in studies to prevent or lower the risk of various chronic diseases to include cancer.[156]

In short, we caution patients with cancer, or a history of cancer, in their gluten consumption. In TCM, gluten can be described in terms of dampness. The symptoms associated with gluten sensitivities and intolerances center around deficiency of the Spleen, but other organs such as the Spleen's pair, the Stomach, as well as the Liver can have diagnostic and therefore therapeutic relevance in treatment. While Western science may not have a definitive connection with gluten and cancer, in TCM, damp and its more concentrated or long-standing form, phlegm, is one of the major pathology patterns associated with cancer. In any chronic disease, the health of the Spleen and Stomach is paramount. Therefore, the issue of damp/phlegm can be pervasive pathogen in neoplastic disease, so it is important to inform patients and create dietary plan that is sustainable and effective.

Should I Do a Fast or Cleanse?

We routinely get asked about fasting and cleansing with our general population of patients, but these questions have become more frequent from our cancer patients over the past two-to-three years. To begin with, any drastic change in diet should be discussed with the primary oncologist and any other healthcare practitioners involved in treatment.

Let's start with the many types of fasting. There are multi-day, whole day, alternate days, and time-restricted, and they usually are either water fasting (water only) or dry fasting (no food or water). Therefore, it is important to clarify which type of fasting the patient is considering. There are various purported benefits with fasting in general, but with respect to cancer, the effects on the body that benefit cancer may include an increase in the production of tumor killing cells, a protective mechanism that protects

---

[156] Dixon, 2013

healthy cells from chemotherapy but not cancer cells and decrease in blood glucose production. These thoughts are largely extrapolated from small studies done on animals such as mice and rats.[157] Otherwise, we are only aware of small case study reports and studies with humans suggesting that fasting could help with chemo-related side-effects and possibly be relatively safe.[158] At this time, our understanding is that the Mayo Clinic is conducting research to investigate the parameters under which fasting may be safely conducted with cancer patients.

It's possible that there is a place for some type of fasting with respect to a preventative approach to cancer. Perhaps it could also be considered appropriate if the patient is otherwise healthy and strong, the cancer was discovered early, or if the patient was very diligent about getting the right nutrition during off-periods of fasting. Typically, the path of health and healing requires the right sufficient nutrition specific to the individual. The approach of cultivating long-term physical strength with nutrient-dense foods can also positively impact one's mental and emotional outlook. This should be taken into consideration with the possibility of recurrence in cancer when long-term health most likely outweighs the benefits of short-term fasting.

In short, we do not advocate fasting for our cancer patients. In TCM, as reflected in *Ling Shu* Chapter 32, prolonged fasting depletes one's *qi*, and if continued will damage one's blood.[159] Some patients ask about practices loosely associated with modern day TCM, such as certain Daoist practices that involve fasting. Our response is that the people taking part in such a practice were probably doing so in conjunction with some degree of seclusion and meditation practice. They weren't fasting while going through chemotherapy, trying to maintain a family and/or job, squeezing in their exercise class, and dealing with the day-to-day stresses that plague modern day lifestyles. Basically, those practices were still focused on conserving energy and not simultaneously expending it.

The concept of dietary cleansing has been around a long time, as a result there are extensive approaches depending on the goal. The primary issue with cleanses is that they are fairly harsh on the body. Flushing the

---

[157] Lee, 2012
[158] Safdie, 2009
[159] Unschuld, 2016

body using herbs or other methods while limiting calories is depleting to one's *qi* and needlessly taxes the body. Even mild juice cleanses still deprive the body of nutrients and add stress to the body. The body already has detoxifying organs such as the Kidney, Liver and Lungs. The easiest way to cleanse is create healthy habits that support these organ system, such as drinking water, eating as clean or organic as possible. Include plenty of fiber, especially cruciferous vegetables, and antioxidants. Also, finding ways to relax and turn-off through meditation and mindfulness practices can have a host of positive, systemic effects on the body.

It's clear that Western nutritional science has accomplished a lot in understanding the therapeutic value of food. Traditional Chinese medicine has incorporated dietary therapy into patient care for thousands of years. Food was the first form of medicine throughout the world. Cancer is a condition that calls for a synergistic aspect to healing over a singular method of approach, which is reflective of integrative oncology values and practices.

References

Aoyagi, T., Terracina, K. P., Raza, A., Matsubara, H., & Takabe, K. (2015). Cancer cachexia, mechanism and treatment. *World Journal of Gastrointestinal Oncology, 7*(4), 17–29. doi:10.4251/wjgo.v7.i4.17

Basta, G., Schmidt, A. M., & De Caterina, R. (2004). Advanced glycation end products and vascular inflammation: Implications for accelerated atherosclerosis in diabetes. Retrieved September 30, 2018, from https://www.ncbi.nlm.nih.gov/pubmed/15306213

Bloomfield, H. E., Koeller, E., Greer, N., MacDonald, R., Kane, R., & Wilt, T. J. (2016). Effects on Health Outcomes of a Mediterranean Diet With No Restriction on Fat Intake: A Systematic Review and Meta-analysis. Retrieved September 20, 2018, from https://www.ncbi.nlm.nih.gov/pubmed/27428849

Cleveland Clinic Cancer Care Team. (2015). The Link Between Red Meat and Cancer: What You Need to Know. Retrieved October 1, 2018, from https://health.clevelandclinic.org/link-red-meat-cancer-need-know/

Coussens, L. M., & Werb, Z. (2002). Inflammation and Cancer [Abstract]. *Nature,* **420**(6917): 860–867. doi:https://doi.org/10.1038/nature01322

Dixon, S. (2013). Does Gluten Cause Cancer? Retrieved September 22, 2018, from https://www.oncologynutrition.org/erfc/hot-topics/does-gluten-cause-cancer/

Dorff, T. B., Groshen, S., Garcia, A., Shah, M., Tsao-Wei, D., Pham, H., Brandhorst, S., Cohen, P., Wei, M., Long, V., Quinn, DI., & Cheng, C. (2016). Safety and Feasibility of Fasting in Combination with Platinum-based Chemotherapy. Retrieved October 3, 2018, from https://bmccancer.biomedcentral.com/articles/10.1186/s12885-016-2370-6

Fernandez, E. (2016). Sugar Papers Reveal Industry Role in Shifting National Heart Disease Focus to Saturated Fat. Retrieved October 5, 2018, from https://www.ucsf.edu/news/2016/09/404081/sugar-papers-reveal-industry-role-shifting-national-heart-disease-focus

Harpaz, D., Yeo, LP., Cecchini, F., et al. (2018). Measuring Artificial Sweeteners Toxicity Using a Bioluminescent Bacterial Panel. Retrieved October 2, 2018, from https://www.ncbi.nlm.nih.gov/pubmed/30257473

Holmes, B. (2015). Chicken Soup for the Aging Star's Soul. Retrieved August 23, 2018, from http://www.espn.com/nba/story/_/id/12168515/bone-broth-soup-helping-los-angeles-lakers-kobe-bryant

Kearns, C. E., Schmidt, L. A., & Glantz, S. A. (2016). Sugar Industry and Coronary Heart Disease Research. Retrieved September 26, 2018, from https://jamanetwork.com/journals/jamainternalmedicine/article-abstract/2548255

Lardieri, A. (2018). Artificial Sweeteners are Toxic to Digestive Gut Bacteria: Study. Retrieved October 4, 2018, from https://www.cnbc.com/2018/10/03/artificial-sweeteners-are-toxic-to-digestive-gut-bacteria-study.html

Lee, C., Raffaghello, L., Brandhorst, S., et al. (2012). Fasting Cycles Retard Growth of Tumors and Sensitize a Range of Cancer Cell Types to Chemotherapy. Retrieved October 5, 2018, from http://stm.sciencemag.org/content/early/2012/02/06/scitranslmed.3003293 DOI: 10.1126/scitranslmed.3003293

Muscaritoli, M., Lucia, S., Farcomeni, A., et al. (2017). Prevalence of Malnutrition in Patients at First Medical Oncology Visit: The PreMiO Study. Retrieved September 29, 2018, from https://www.ncbi.nlm.nih.gov/pmc/articles/PMC5668103/

National Cancer Institute. (2017). Nutrition in Cancer Care. Retrieved September 27, 2018, from https://www.cancer.gov/about-cancer/treatment/side-effects/appetite-loss/nutrition-hp-pdq#cit/section_1.11

Prado, S. B., Ferreira, G. F., Harazono, Y., Shiga, T. M., Raz, A., Carpita, N. C., & Fabi, J. P. (2017). Ripening-induced Chemical Modifications of Papaya Pectin Inhibit Cancer Cell Proliferation. Retrieved October 1, 2018, from https://www.nature.com/articles/s41598-017-16709-3

Rocha, N. S., Barbisan, L. F., De Oliveira, M. L., & De Camargo, J. L. (2002). Effects of Fasting and Intermittent Fasting on Rat Hepatocarcinogenesis Induced by

Diethylnitrosamine. Retrieved October 5, 2018, from https://www.ncbi.nlm.nih.gov/pubmed/11835290

Roepe, L. R. (2018). The Diet Industry. Retrieved August 15, 2018, from http://businessresearcher.sagepub.com/sbr-1946-105904-2881576/20180305/the-diet-industry

Safdie, F. M., Dorff, T., Quinn, D., Fontana, L., Wei, M., Lee, C., Cohen, P., & Longo, V. D. (2009). Fasting and Cancer Treatment in Humans: A Case Series Report. Retrieved September 23, 2018, from https://www.ncbi.nlm.nih.gov/pmc/articles/PMC2815756/

Tontonoz, M. (2016). Memorial Sloan Kettering Cancer Center: No Sugar, No Cancer? A Look at the Evidence. Retrieved October 2, 2018, from https://www.mskcc.org/blog/no-sugar-no-cancer-look-evidence

Tontonoz, M. (2016). No Sugar, No Cancer? A Look at the Evidence. Retrieved October 2, 2018, from https://www.mskcc.org/blog/no-sugar-no-cancer-look-evidence

Torgan, C. (2018). Food Additives Alter Gut Microbes, Cause Diseases in Mice. Retrieved August 22, 2018, from https://www.nih.gov/news-events/nih-research-matters/food-additives-alter-gut-microbes-cause-diseases-mice

Unschuld, P. U. (Trans.). (2016). *Huang Di Nei Jing Ling Shu — the Ancient Classic on Needle Therapy*. Oakland, CA: University Of California Press.

Willett, W. C. (2000). Diet and Cancer. The Oncologist, 5(5), 393–404. doi:10.1634/theoncologist.5-5-393

World Cancer Research Fund. (2018). Limit Red and Processed Meat. Retrieved September 29, 2018, from https://www.wcrf.org/dietandcancer/recommendations/limit-red-processed-meat

World Health Organization. (2015). Q&A on the Carcinogenicity of the Consumption of Red Meat and Processed Meat. Retrieved September 26, 2018, from https://www.iarc.fr/en/media-centre/iarcnews/pdf/Monographs-Q&A_Vol114.pdf

Zhang, Y., Wan, Y., Huo, B., Li, B., Jin, Y., & Hu, X. (2018). Extracts and Components of Ficus Carica Leaves Suppress Survival, Cell Cycle, and Migration of Triple-Negative Breast Cancer MDA-MB-231 Cells. Retrieved September 24, 2018, from https://www.ncbi.nlm.nih.gov/pmc/articles/PMC6067789/

8 Eight Extraordinary Meridians

"We can study until old age ... and still not finish."

Chinese Proverb

Chinese medicine examines disease through an organized system of theory and principles. This allows the practitioner to interpret multifactorial presentations, such as cancer, within an established framework. What developed from thousands of years of empirical evidence by Chinese scholars was a method of analysis recognized as systematic correspondence. The theory contends that most or even all phenomena, which includes natural occurrences and abstract concepts, can be incorporated into a correlated system that came to dominate Chinese medico-theoretical literature.[160] It identifies a mutual dependence and conversely mutual influence with occurrences (phenomena), both in the body and the natural world, through an inherent parallel with particular avenues of conformity. This applies both in an individual's body, with respect to their state of health or disease, including the physical and mental-emotional, but also with one's relationship to the outside world and environment. In TCM, this method of understanding can be applied both diagnostically and therapeutically.

It is with this introduction we enter into the esoteric therapy of the eight extraordinary meridians (EEM) for cancer management, one of the more complex and least understood aspects of traditional Chinese medicine. Its therapeutic range addresses the physical, mental-emotional, congenital

---

[160] Unschuld, 1985

and even spiritual aspect of a person, something desperately needed by cancer patients. Of all the techniques and modalities, it is the eight extras that have yielded profound results because of its innate ability to access these elements. However, experience indicates this intricate system is not well understood by clinicians, and perhaps, this is why it is not often applied in clinical practice. Fortunately, much of the understanding and relevance of the EEM is being rediscovered by modern day scholars. As is true for much of Chinese medicine history, the act of burning books during dynasty changes in an attempt to erase whole swaths of history certainly affected sharing of information. The most recent destruction of material occurred under the rule of Mao Tse-tung. Despite crediting TCM for the role it played in treating his soldiers through their victory, he dismissed traditional practices in favor of Western medicine. As a consequence, many doctors, carriers of historical medicine passed down among generations, fled or were driven out of the country. Thus, a potential treasure-trove of information and experience was lost to history, including the EEM. This has left the task of rediscovery to modern practitioners, and the timing could not be better. The potency of eight extra treatments during the cancer journey unveils an immense terrain of healing that is both empowering and nurturing for the patient.

Thus, complex disease patterns and mental-emotional conditions may rely upon the EEM to deliver results. With this approach, the practitioner works with a patient's *jing*, or essence. This is different from treating the more superficial *qi* and blood aspect through regular meridians, which invokes strong physical-emotional sensations that can be relatively short-lived. This is reflective when patients demonstrate a reduction in pain or stress for a few days, but it slowly returns within the week. By comparison, essence lies deeper in the body and as such, it is thought to move much slower than *qi* and blood. The effects at the time of treatment can be described as subtle, but its energy is more long-lasting and unfolds over a longer period of time. By virtue of the physiological functions of each of the eight meridians, there is a vast degree of potential to influence life changes, propel decision-making, reconnect to the true self and imbue the physical body with deeper levels of relief. It is a unique system that embodies a multifaceted approach, and in doing so, connects the individual to the energy needed at the time of treatment.

It is important to note that the relative intensity of these treatments has an effect in the hours, days and even weeks after treatment and therefore, extensive application is cautioned. Some scholars even argue that the eight extras should never be utilized because they deal with a patient's *essence*. This may be related to differing interpretations of classical texts, or from medical history that claims this form of treatment was banned in China for a few hundred years because it was thought to be so powerful it could change a person's destiny. According to a lecture delivered by Jeffrey Yuen in 2004 at the Swedish Institute, it was not until the Ming Dynasty (1368–1644 A.D.) that the EEM treatments even became popular. Prior to this time period, it was considered inappropriate to utilize the EEM because of their influence on the constitutional level potentially altering a person's destiny.[161] This implied that treatments could affect congenital issues directly. Modern analyses by Chinese medicine scholars correlate this theory to the potential influence with regard to genetic mutations and actually changing one's DNA and RNA.[162] It is more likely the possibility of affecting the expression of DNA, an interesting concept with respect to the cellular level of cancer pathology.[163]

The aforementioned system of correspondence is at the core of this technique. It is a dualistic concept, much like *yin* and *yang*, two opposite yet complementary categories that reflect a basic interdependence. Conversely, it is thought by many to be the highest form of Chinese medicine. By incorporating this system into practice, a practitioner accesses the core framework of an individual, one's identity and understanding of self.[164] It is similar to a braided rope in that each strand can be unraveled from the others, but when intertwined the rope is strong and complete. The physicality of a cancer diagnosis certainly merits treatment to reduce physical discomfort. However, when issues arise that cannot be relieved by meridian treatments or physical medicine, the practitioner must address the root and turn to the EEM. This method integrates the individual's experiences. When this occurs, the body integrates on a physical, mental-emotional and spiritual level to

---

[161] Isabella, 2004
[162] ibid
[163] Frost, 2010
[164] ibid

achieve balance. Ideally this leads toward deep, meaningful and lasting healing and ultimately enhances the body's own natural ability to heal itself.

Historical perspective is certainly warranted on such an intriguing from of medicine. The section that follows illuminates the path of EEM in Chinese medicine's rich history. Once established, the chapter evolves into application and treatment. This enables the TCM practitioner to explore the dynamics of this approach for cancer patients. The following pages are not an exhaustive review of this unique system. This section is intended to provide the licensed acupuncture practitioner or committed student of Chinese medicine with academic information and clinical perspective to build upon. For those reading who are unfamiliar with TCM, it offers an interesting glimpse into the more esoteric, yet clinically relevant side of the medicine.

A Brief History of Eight Extra Meridians

Li Shi-Zhen once said, "If physicians are not aware of such theories of the extraordinary channels, they will remain in the dark as to the cause of disease."[165] It's likely that oral tradition, including early debate and transmission of knowledge about the EEM, existed long before anyone decided to start writing it down. It is unclear where in the progression and development of Chinese medicine that the EEM were discovered and initially established. In early Han Dynasty (206 B.C.–220 A.D.), some of the earliest texts, specifically *Basic Questions* and *Divine Pivot*, already argued that the twelve primary channels and extraordinary meridians were intertwined. These texts presented the EEM as regulators of the entire channel system by means of governing the overall balance of *yin* and *yang*.[166] In the seminal text, *Classic of Difficulties*, which is thought to be written in the late Han Dynasty, the function of the extraordinary meridians was thought to absorb the overflow of *qi* from the primary meridians. Thus, *qi* could flow into, but not out of, the extraordinary meridians.[167] The understanding of the EEM continued to evolve with the development of the opening points by Xu Feng in his book

---

[165] Chace & Shima, 2010
[166] ibid
[167] ibid

Comprehensive Compendium of Acupuncture and Moxibustion based on the holes first identified by Dou Han-Qing in 1196 A.D.[168]

Li Shi-Zhen's *Qi Jing Ba Mai Gao* is arguably the most important, or perhaps the most influential volume of the eight extraordinary meridians. This text is a compilation of tenets and practices according to previously written manuscripts presenting EEM and internal alchemy. He emphasized pulse technique associated with each extra meridian and challenged the concept of opening points that correspond to the channel. Li Shi-Zhen believed it unnecessary to needle opening point(s) to access an extra meridian and instead treat along the trajectory of the channel. This is contrary to modern teachings of EEM technique that instructs practitioners to begin with the opening point. However, perhaps due to his affinity for the *Inner Classic and Pulse Classic*, he ascertained the use of locations outside the channel as a method to activate the extraordinary meridians. This is one of his less accepted ideas and could be due to the fact he modified the pathways of the extraordinary meridians and described them in much greater detail than had been previously written.

Regardless, Li Shi-Zhen's contributions to the theory and application of EEM are well accepted. He conveyed an instrumental idea between the relationship of the extraordinary meridians and the primary channels: a reciprocal flow of *qi*. Specifically, Li Shi-Zhen said, "The overflow of *qi* [from the channels and networks] enters the extraordinary vessels providing reciprocal irrigation, internally warming the viscera and receptacles, and externally moistening the interstices."[169] This was a vast difference from the *Classic of Difficulties'* stance on the role of the EEM in the body and fundamentally changed the view of how these meridians address the pathogenesis of disease and influence treatment.

Basic Development and Concepts of the Eight Extras

The innate composition of the eight extras is formed at conception. The *jing* from the female and male energy combine to form the *Chong* channel.

---

[168] Cecil-Sturman, 2012
[169] Chase et al., 2010

From this primary pathway, the *Ren* and *Du* meridians unfold. The *Wei* and *Qiao* channels follow to nearly complete the human form. The *Dai* meridian evolves from these established channels and completes the energetic body. This pattern is an imprint upon each individual similar to a genetic code. This intrinsic connection to one's development at conception, combined with the traits inherited from the female and male body, enable the treatment of physical injury, complex illnesses and mental-emotional conditions. Of these, it is well-established that principles of TCM and acupuncture specifically can alleviate physical ailments. It is equally understood that these manifestations are expressions of internal disharmony and stuck emotions. Humans, afterall, are creatures that inherently embody complex thought and emotion. Critical thinking and the compassionate heart has inspired the evolutionary process.

Chinese medicine is remarkable at treating the Heart or *shen* for acute symptoms as a result of mental-emotional imbalance. When events occur that deeply penetrate an individual, that break through all defenses, there is a shift within the physical, mental and emotional self. The response is uniquely physiological to the constitution. The emotional terrain is inherently linked to the genetic traits from which they are created. To summarize the capacity and depth of these channels, Penn Chiao, author of the *Nan Jing* writes, "Only those who master the eight extraordinary vessels, besides the twelve major meridians, can make a correct diagnosis, and only those who know how to use the extraordinary vessels can eradicate the illness, which is often deeper than one thinks."[170]

The idea that the twelve primary channels are separate from the EEM originally came from the 27th Difficult Issue in the *Classic of Difficulties*.[171] As noted, the EEM do not have the same internal-external pairing as the twelve primary meridians. Aside from the *Wei* vessel's connection to the concept of protective or *wei qi*, the EEM do not relate to external influences like the twelve primary meridians. Consequently, they are considered as the inner organization of life and actually prepare the pathway for the twelve regular meridians of the adult.[172] Other differences include the fact that the EEM are not associated with any *zang-fu* and do not have points of their own but are actually accessed through regular meridian points. Because the

---

[170] Frost, 2010
[171] Chace et al., 2010
[172] Rochat De La Vallee, 1997

energy that flows through these extraordinary channels is *jing* and *yuan qi*, versus the *zheng qi* in the twelve meridians, it tends to flow more slowly. Thus the treatment duration is longer in order to allow this subtle energy to circulate. We allow 40–45 minutes, as opposed to the 20 minutes commonly thought to be sufficient for regular meridian treatments.

Classically, the functions of the EEM can be summarized as reservoirs for *qi* with the purpose of absorbing excess *qi* from the primary meridians. This *qi* is returned back to the main channels that exhibit deficiency. The eight extras protect against evil *qi*, regulate the changes of the life cycle that occurs at seven-year intervals for women and eight-year intervals for men and circulate the *jing* (essence) to the entire body including the six extraordinary organs: Brain, Marrow (spine and bone marrow), Gall Bladder, Uterus, Blood Vessels and Bone. Modern clinical specialists of this method have added a tremendous amount of philosophical thought and practical application over the years. Two of the more prominent scholars at the forefront of the continued development of the understanding of the EEM are Mark Frost, Professor at the American College of Traditional Chinese Medicine and Jeffrey Yuen whose body of knowledge is reflected in his student Ann Cecil-Sterman's book *Advanced Acupuncture a Clinic Manual*. In order to clearly delineate the immense therapeutic value of these meridians, refer to the outline below that highlights key properties and functions. Except where noted, the following replicates notes that were taken in a class taught by Professor Mark Frost in 2010, which reflects his more than 20 years of modern EEM clinical experience.

Properties of EEM

- There is no specific organ associated with the channels. However, they treat conditions from specific organs, like *Chong* and *Ren* for the Uterus, *Chong* for the Heart, etc.
- Each extra meridian has a master or confluent point, a point to enliven that specific meridian. Think of it as a light switch. You turn the switch on the wall on, rather than screwing in a light bulb, and the whole system lights up.

(Continued)

---

[173] Chase et al., 2010

(Continued)

Properties of EEM

- The *Ren, Du, Chong* and *Dai* all have the same origin, arising from the same location in the body, the *Bao Zhong*, also known as the Gestational Membrane.[173] For those unfamiliar with TCM, this is described as being in the lower *dan tian*, or roughly a couple finger widths below the navel.
- The *qi* does not flow in a particular direction in the EEM, rather the movement of *qi* is like the tide; it does not circulate from A to B, but rhythmically ebbs and flows in a tide-like quality.
- *Jing qi* circulates in these meridians, rather than *zheng qi* (true *qi*).
- Tonification or sedation is not applied on any of the points because *jing qi* does not require manipulation. Although this theory is debated in modern times, classical thought dictates the points are opened, accessed it and left.
- Excluding the *Ren* and *Du*, there are not specific points along the EEM.
- The names of the EEM indicate their function whereas the names of regular meridians indicate their source and influence with respect to the organ the channel is associated with. For example, within the name *Yin Wei Mai* — *wei* means gathering or linking, therefore this is a meridian that gathers or links the *yin*.

Functions of the EEM

- Coordinate and link the *shen* of the body to facilitate a smooth integration of the *shen*. Provide a bridge between the physical and the non-physical bodies.
- Provide the mechanism by which heaven enters into earth allowing the primordial *qi* (pure consciousness) to enter the human being.
- Absorb excess *qi*. The channels offer a release valve or a reservoir, so the regular meridians have an outflow excess energy.
- Maintain homeostasis. Absorb excess and provide in a state of insufficiency.
- Counteract evil *qi*. Toxic events from the past can be sequestered away and start to rise up like an infection, releasing its toxic content.

(Continued)

Functions of the EEM

- Regulate the life cycles, by ruling the seven- and eight-year cycles that determine development and maturation for women and men respectively. Essentially signposts of growth from birth to old age. Includes regulation of the hormonal cycles and function.

- Responsible for the circulation of the *jing qi* and the practical expression of *yuan qi*. The active component of the ancestral energy stored in the *Bao Zhong* (*dan tian*).

- Circulate and express protective *wei qi*. Primal role in counteracting *du qi* (toxic *qi*). Excess sexual activity followed by exposure to toxic *qi* will permeate the body very deeply. The *wei qi* will be affected and weakened.

- Address congenital or constitutional problems, which have the capacity to influence our developmental expression. For example, weakness of the adrenal or thyroid glands, developmental issues in children.

- Profoundly useful in addressing endocrine problems. *Du* meridian for adrenal exhaustion, and/or thyroid function; *Yin Wei* for low estrogenic function, boosting *yin*, addressing menopausal conditions.

- Emotional and psychological issues are accessed by these channels to treat the spirit or *shen*; unresolved issues of the past reside in the extraordinary vessels.

- Spiritual transformation. Supports movement toward the final unique purpose of life, moving toward knowing one's own essence, the ancestor of the one unique *qi*, according to Daoist alchemy and spiritual transformation.

Many indications can be extrapolated from the properties and functions of the EEM. Its therapeutic scope encompasses the whole person, the physical, mental-emotional, energetic and spiritual core. By accessing these channels, the energy of the body is optimized to remove blockages that inhibit restored health. This encourages the true self to integrate meaningful thoughts and emotions into a more profound healing realm. The synergy of EEM with supportive TCM modalities, such as moxibustion and herbal medicine, also restore the body and mind. This seamless integration integrates in a manner that empowers a patient to focus on their capacity for self-healing.

The following section is a general overview presenting the discourse of each extraordinary meridian. The intent is to offer an exposition of this unique system that demonstrates its multifaceted scope in cancer care. This is relevant for TCM clinicians who have the necessary foundation and skills to implement the eight extras in practice, as well as the general reader curious about the breadth of therapies that Chinese medicine can provide.

The *Chong* channel

Opening Point: SP-4 (*gong sun*)
Coupled Point: PC-6 (*nei guan*)

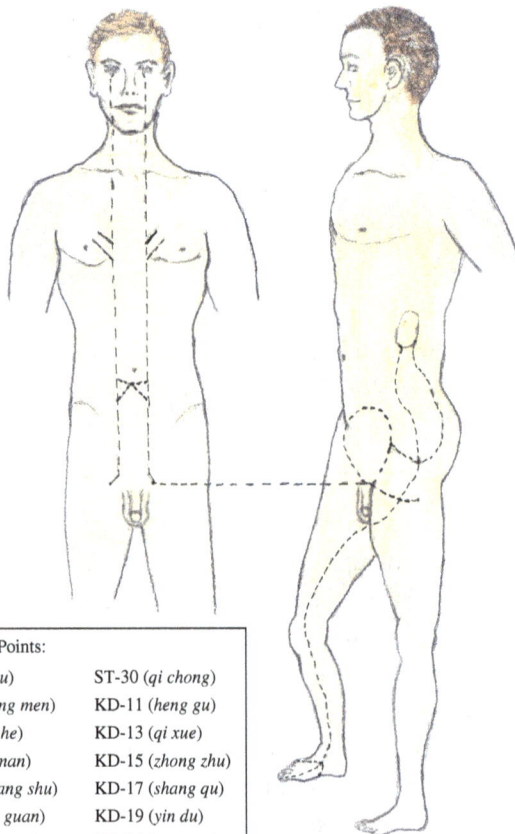

Trajectory Points:

CV-2 (*qu gu*)	ST-30 (*qi chong*)
SP-12 (*chong men*)	KD-11 (*heng gu*)
KD-12 (*da he*)	KD-13 (*qi xue*)
KD-14 (*si man*)	KD-15 (*zhong zhu*)
KD-16 (*huang shu*)	KD-17 (*shang qu*)
KD-18 (*shi guan*)	KD-19 (*yin du*)
KD-20 (*tong gu*)	KD-21 (*you men*)

Functions: The basic functions of the *Chong* are the storage and dissemination of blood and source *qi* to regulate the channels and vessels.[174] The *Chong* meridian is known as the "Sea of the Twelve Channels", taking this name from an internal branch that travels up the inside of the spine and defining an axis by which all the channels are aligned. It is also this connection that leaves it vulnerable to become out of balance by the means of any channel.[175] The *Chong* is the deepest vessel in the body and can be thought of as the interior boundary for all the channels. This meridian imposes its influence from the inside outward and maintains a longitudinal regulation of the channels.

Along with the *Ren* and *Du* meridians, the *Chong* has a close association with the moving *qi*, or source *qi*, between the Kidneys. It is this relationship with source *qi* that connects the *Chong* and the *San Jiao*, the channel that transmits source *qi* in the body. The Spleen and Liver are also linked to the *Chong* along with the Kidney, as referenced.

Pathophysiology: Disease can be described by two core pathological mechanisms, counterflow and abdominal urgency.[176] Examples of counterflow include headache and dizziness, fainting and syncope, wheezing and difficulty catching one's breath. Abdominal urgency can include issues related to pain, distention and discomfort. As well, with all EEM, pathologies can include issues that arise along the trajectory of the meridian. From a mental-emotional level, the *Chong* is about the self, 'Who am I?' perceiving a person's deepest experience of self.[177] It helps a person discern which of their mental-emotional responses are from their true nature versus which responses are developed from social or familial conditioning.[178] Of note, from a physical diagnostic standpoint, palpation of the abdominal aortic pulse in the lower left quadrant can be indicative of a *Chong* dysfunction.

Chong and Cancer: The *Chong* is frequently incorporated into our treatments for cancer patients. It is particularly effective for cancer-related symptoms; those that are physical as well as emotional. *Chong* is known as the "Sea of

---

[174] Chace et al., 2010
[175] ibid
[176] Chace et al., 2010
[177] Frost, 2010
[178] Cecil-Sterman, 2012

Blood" and is therefore indicated for blood deficient patterns because of its ability to tonify blood. Chinese medicine theory correlates blood vacuity to many factors, including lifestyle, poor diet, overwork and longstanding illness. Thus, blood deficient patterns predispose a constitution to pathogenic invasion. In terms of neoplastic disease, blood deficiency is perpetuated by conventional medicine therapies such as cytotoxic medicine, radiation and pharmaceutical drugs. Thus, it becomes a cyclical condition that is present at every phase of cancer, from early to end stage. Another feature associated with the *Chong* meridian as the "Sea of Blood" is its ability to move blood throughout the body. This is integral for pain relief, inflammation and stagnation as it generates circulation to alleviate areas of physical congestion.

Perhaps the most therapeutic aspect of the *Chong* is its ability to reacquaint an individual with their true self, who they are in the deepest, purest sense. The *Chong* is the very basis of the human spirit. Even before the physical body forms at conception, the energetic body takes shape and the *Chong* develops. In the complexity of cancer management, it is a frequent occurrence to observe patients who have "lost themselves" and solely identify with their disease and diagnosis. This presentation is quite individualized, but we have observed this disconnect from self with patients who have just received a cancer diagnosis, already undone, or mid-late stage patients who have in a sense, given up. The *Chong* can realign the energy of the body with the spirit in a restorative sense. While this does not alter the prognosis, we have observed profound changes in attitude that restore optimism. The simplicity of this treatment is a true integration of the emotional terrain relative to life experiences, health and well-being.

General Physiological and Psychological Conditions Associated with the Chong

Long-term Spleen *qi* deficiency	Lower abdomen damp-heat and leakage as seen in Irritable Bowel Syndrome (IBS), Crohn's disease, ulcerative colitis	Addison's disease

(Continued)

General Physiological and Psychological Conditions Associated with the Chong

Five *zang* accumulations: Heart, the hidden beam; Spleen, abdominal focal distention; Lung, dyspnea; Kidney, running piglet *qi*; and Liver, fatty deposits	The five jaundices resulting from food poisoning, hepatitis, alcohol, excess sex, and limbic	Heart pain, with fullness and knotting behind or below the sternum
Blood stasis: systemic and especially the Heart and Liver	Splenomegaly	*Bi* syndrome. Intractable pain in joints, stiff lower back, disc herniation, fractures, blockage of the sensory orifices
Difficulty relaxing or concentration	Anxiety and panic attacks	Chronic fatigue with depression
Insomnia	Digestive disorders, including diarrhea and food stasis	Nausea, vomiting and esophageal reflux
Knotted chest (chest pain)	Gynecological conditions: irregular menses, dysmenorrhea, fibroids, endometriosis, yeast infections and leucorrhea, miscarriage, and hot flashes	Urogenital conditions and prostatitis
Hypertension from renal insufficiency	Dwarfism and being small for one's age	Postural issues from *yang* deficiency
Alzheimer's and dementia	Physical and/or mental exhaustion	

(Continued)

(Continued)

Physiological Indications of the *Chong* Channel from Professor Mark Frost	
Peripheral vascular disorders	Cardiovascular disease such as angina and atrial fibrillation
Dysuria and anuria	Placental retention
Edema	

Psychological Indications of the *Chong* channel included from Ann Cecil-Sterman:[179]	
Shen imbalance	Birth trauma
Unmet physiological and emotional needs since birth	Lacking sense of self; not able to feel nourished within one's self; poor self-perception in the present moment

Psychological Indications of the *Chong* Channel included from Ann Cecil-Sterman:	
Aid in the discovery of a person's true nature	Aid in the determination of which of their habitual responses are the product of social or familial conditioning and which are born of their true nature
Aid people to understand who they really are and to help access their deepest desires so that one can know how to achieve fulfillment in life	Discomfort with one's ethnic, racial, and/or cultural identity, discomfort with one's gender and/or sexual identity
Failure of the child to walk by age two or desire in a child to walk too early before they have the capability	Psychosomatic panic attacks
Being able to mentally keep things in place	

---

[179] Cecil-Sterman, 2012

(Continued)

Additional Psychological Indications from Professor Mark Frost	
Depression, feeling "stuck" in life, not moving forward in life	To help a person known themselves better. *Chong* connects directly to our highest self/universal self
To clarify the meaning of this moment in one's life	At times of critical transformation in life — threshold moments, or grand transitions
To help a person clarify their long-term view of life: their purpose, calling, or dharma	

The *Ren* channel

Opening Point: LU-7 (*lie que*)
Coupled Point: KD-6 (*zhao hai*)

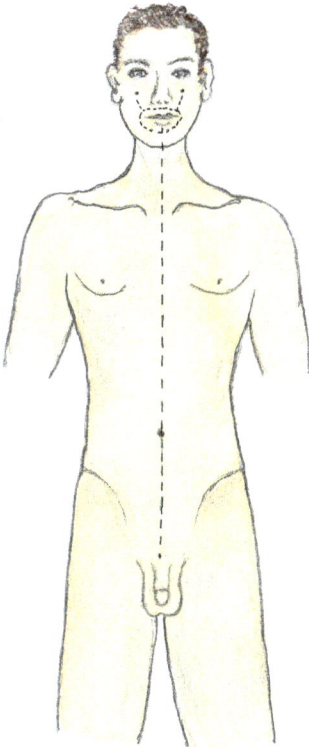

Trajectory Points:

Begins behind CV-3 (*zhong ji*)

then CV-1 (*hui yin*) CV-2 (*qu gu*)

CV-3 (*zhong ji*)	CV-4 (*guan yuan*)
CV-5 (*shi men*)	CV-6 (*qi hai*)
CV-7 (*yin jiao*)	CV-8 (*shen que*)
CV-9 (*shui fen*)	CV-10 (*xia wan*)
CV-11 (*jian li*)	CV-12 (*zhong wan*)
CV-13 (*shang wan*)	CV-14 (*ju que*)
CV-15 (*jiuwei*)	CV-16 (*zhong ting*)
CV-17 (*shan zhong*)	CV-18 (*yu tang*)
CV-19 (*zi gong*)	CV-20 (*hua gai*)
CV-21 (*xuan ji*)	CV-22 (*tian tu*)
CV-23 (*lian quan*)	CV-24 (*cheng jiang*)
ST-4 (*di cang*)	ST-1 (*cheng qi*)

Functions: The *Ren* channel is known as the "Sea of *Yin*" because it is the fundamental manager of *yin* in the body. Whereas the *Chong* regulates blood in the body, the *Ren* is responsible for the movement of *qi* and fluids, especially the proper distribution of *yin* substances and meridians. The *Ren* is often associated with the feminine mother. Traditionally, mothers have a role of nourishing the family but also maintain certain aspects of order as well. This concept can be likened to the differences between the *Chong* and *Ren*. Whereas the *Chong* is more regulatory of blood in the body, the *Ren* regulates *qi* and fluids in order to properly distribute *yin* substances throughout the body. Thus, it is nourishing and circulating. This governing aspect of the *Ren* correlates to its regulation of the life cycles in TCM, of seven years for women and eight years for men.

Pathophysiology: Due to its pathway, the *Ren* is affected by respiratory, digestive, and urogenital issues. Classical pathology is most closely associated with bulging disorders in men, characterized by swelling or pain in the scrotum or abdomen, and vaginal discharge, mobile abdominal masses and gatherings in women. These can be succinctly characterized as internal clumping.[180] These forms of accumulation may equate to what we now identify as tumors, which occur along the pathway of the channel. Modern interpretations of *Ren* pathology include issues with the endocrine system and hormonal regulation.[181] On a mental-emotional level, the *Ren* is affected by the reciprocal bond between a mother and child and treats issues relating to bonding, such as lack of bonding or extensive attachment. In addition, difficulty receiving love and support, as well as a lack of life satisfaction are psycho-emotional indications that calls for a *Ren* treatment.

Ren and Cancer: The *Ren* is a compelling meridian that may not be the first EEM considered for cancer-related conditions, but it does have remarkable features that merits its usage. The channel courses through the midline of the body, much like a zipper. As such, it traverses through

---

[180] Chase et al., 2010
[181] Frost, 2010

three core aspects: the pelvis, abdomen and chest. This correlates to the grouping of organs that are characterized within the TCM concept of the three *jiao*. The lower *jiao* corresponds to the pelvis and its related organs of the urogenital system. Thus cancers that affect this area, like uterine, cervical and bladder can be treated with the *Ren*. The middle *jiao* encompasses the gastrointestinal system, and thus the *Ren* can address pathology related to gastric cancers of the stomach and colon, or of the liver and pancreas. The chest comprises the upper *jiao* and includes the breasts, lungs, heart and esophagus.

An example of a *Ren* treatment is demonstrated in a case with a 46-year-old woman diagnosed with stage II breast cancer. A steady history of issues with her mother demonstrated complex emotional dynamics related to bonding and general dissatisfaction in life. The combination of the *Ren's* ability to access physical imbalance in the upper body and its therapeutic quality, indicated its usage. This treatment was balanced with the *Chong* to also incorporate blood moving aspects to support her body's physical response to surgery and chemotherapy.

Physiological Indications of the Ren channel			
Buffalo hump	Club fingers and toes	Fibroids, endo-metriosis and ovarian cysts	Tumors
Scrotal swell-ings, and testicular pain	Genital dysfunction	Chest oppression	Valve or sphincter issues, including issues with the heart, digestion and respiration
Difficulty swal-lowing	Dryness	Back pain with profuse sweating and straight-ening of the lumbar region	

(Continued)

(Continued)

Additional Physiological Indications from Professor Mark Frost

Delayed puberty	Menopause and early menopause	Withdrawal from opiates and resulting over excitation of the central nervous system
Infertility due to deficiency or *qi* stagnation	Menstrual issues	

Psychological Indications of the *Ren* Meridian from Cecil-Sterman[182]

Difficult bonding to the breast of the mother	Resistance to early weaning	Difficulty or fear of commitment	Habitually forming inappropriate relationships	Feeling incomplete or something is missing
Dependence & over-dependence issues	Tendency to control or be controlled in relationships	Feeling disconnected/ unconnected	Tendency to feel victimized	Inability to feel comfortable responding to people

Psychological Indications of the *Ren* Meridian from Cecil-Sterman

Neediness	Lack of independence	Preference for being pampered	Inability to make decisions for one's self	Inability to connect with anyone
Addictions	Difficulty with understanding one's identity	Feeling incomplete in the absence of a partner	Always wanting something in the mouth, addiction to talking	Bulimia

---

182 Cecil-Sterman, 2012

The *Du* channel

Opening Point: SI-3 (*hou xi*)
Coupled Point: UB-62 (*shen mai*)

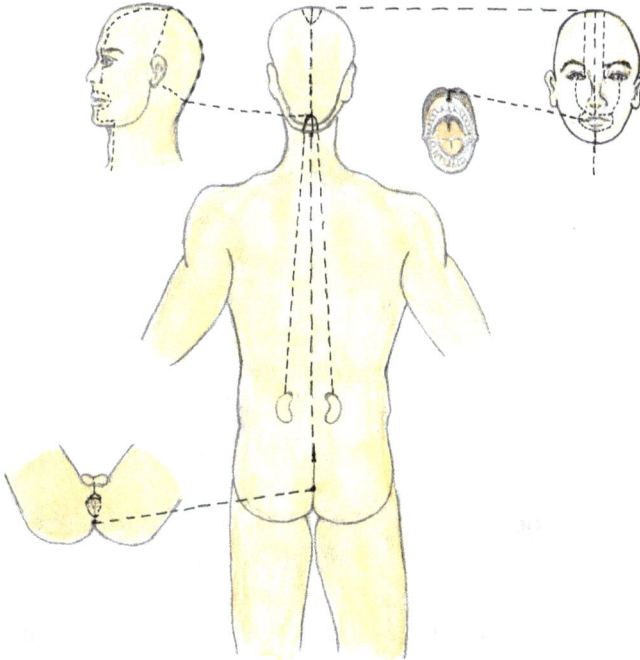

Trajectory Points:			
Channel begins beneath the pole *(xia ji)*			
GV-1 *(hang qiang)*	GV-2 *(yaos hu)*	GV-15 *(ya men)*	GV-16 *(fengfu)*
GV-3 *(yao yang guan)*	GV-4 *(ming men)*	GV-17 *(naohu)*	GV-18 *(qiang jian)*
GV-5 *(xuan shu)*	GV-6 *(ji zhong)*	GV-19 *(hou ding)*	GV-20 *(bai hui)*
GV-7 *(zhong shu)*	GV-8 *(jin suo)*	GV-21 *(qian ding)*	GV-22 *(xin hui)*
GV-9 *(zhi yang)*	GV-10 *(ling tai)*	GV-23 *(shang xing)*	GV-24 *(shenting)*
GV-11 *(shen dao)*	GV-12 *(shen zhu)*	GV-25 *(su liao)*	GV-26 *(ren zhong)*
GV-13 *(tao dao)*	GV-14 *(da zhui)*	GV-27 *(dui duan)*	GV-28 *(yin jiao)*

Functions: The *Du* meridian is known as the "Sea of *Yang*." Its energetic pair is the lower abdomen, "Sea of *Yin*." Both are considered sources for the activation of primordial *yang*.[183] *Du Mai* is also called the Governing Vessel

---

[183] Chase et al., 2010

because it governs, or controls, all the *yang* meridians in the body. *Yang* has many characteristics in TCM, but a few of them include: generating, action, energy, rising, expansion and function. These traits combine with the pathway of the channel through the central nervous system (CNS) to reveal many of the pathophysiological and metaphysical involvements of the *Du*. This includes growth and development, immunity, mental stagnation, exhaustion (physical, mental, emotional, spiritual) and inflammatory conditions. The *Du's* pathway and connection in the body makes it one of the best to treat physical issues and the body's overall functioning. If *yin* is the material of life, then *yang* is the force that puts it in action.

In trying to bridge the gap between the TCM understanding of the body compared to Western medicine, we can break down some of the *Du's* functions and influence on the body by looking at some of the important anatomical connections. The *Du* is associated with the central nervous system and endocrine function because of its pathway up through the spine and into the brain. Likewise, because it enters the brain at the base of the occiput at *DU-16* (*feng fu*) and exits at the vertex *DU-20* (*bai hui*), it has a far-reaching effect on the physical to the mental-emotional and reflects why *DU-20* (*bai hui*) is called "one hundred convergences." Major glands of the body, such as the pituitary, pineal and adrenals are connected to the *Du* by virtue of its pathway as well as its inherent connection to the Kidneys. This integrative perspective offers compelling information that enforces a dualistic approach to pathophysiology and treatment as illustrated in the following conceptual framework:

Gland	Biomedicine	Chinese Medicine
Hypothalamus	Hormonal regulation, growth and development, appetite, emotional responses	Seven- and eight-year cycles for men and women EEM: *Du, Chong, Dai* Primary: Kidney, Spleen, Liver
Thalamus	Regulates sleep, relay motor-sensory (auditory, visual, tactile) signals to cerebral cortex	EEM: *Du, Yin Wei, Yang Wei, Yang Qiao* Primary: Kidney, Heart, Liver, Spleen
Pineal	Production and regulation of melatonin for sleep regulation[184]	EEM: *Du, Yin Wei, Chong* Primary: Liver, Heart, Kidney

Pituitary	Considered the "master gland," part of endocrine system that secretes hormones that affect reproductive organs, thyroid and adrenals	EEM: *Du, Ren, Chong* Primary: Spleen, Kidney, Heart
Endocrine system	Metabolism, growth, sexual development and function	EEM: *Du, Ren, Chong* Primary: Kidney, Spleen

Pathophysiology: As with all meridians, pain, stiffness and spasm can present along the channel. Orthopedic complaints that include spinal vertebrae, disc issues, and their associated musculature correspond to this meridian. Other classical pathological manifestations include heart pain that affects ability to urinate or defecate, infertility, dribbling urine and blockage, urinary frequency, dry throat, arched-back rigidity contractures and heavy headedness with inability to hold it up.[185] On a mental-emotional level, when the *Du* meridian is balanced, a person feels independent and free and does not have trouble moving forward in life. When it is out of balance, there can be a lack of independence, an inability to move forward, or the opposite can manifest in the form of rebellion.[186]

Du and Cancer: The *Du Mai* is extremely beneficial for cancer support because of its influence on immunity and ability to tonify *yang*. A principle pattern in late stage cancer is *yang* depletion, particularly after an extended battle with the disease and often as a consequence of allopathic medicine. For instance, radiation and certain chemotherapeutic drugs can cause excess heat that damages the *yin* leading to vacuity patterns with heat toxicity. The pathogenic heat will also engender the *yang* to an extent that it burns out. The result is *yin* and *yang* depletion, also known as *essence* deficiency. This phase warrants close attention because it leads toward a path of serious decline and a separation of *yin* and *yang*.

---

[184] Recent studies are examining the impediment of the pineal gland and an increase in cancer risk, such as a 2015 report on a study done on rats (Frajacomo, 2015), as well as the anticancer effects of melatonin (Bella, 2013).

[185] Chase et al., 2010

[186] Cecil-Sterman, 2012

It is during this period, clinicians must assess the degree of fatigue as reported by the patient and through diagnostic inquiry. There are a myriad of signs and symptoms that demonstrate *yang* deficiency is becoming more pronounced. In *qi* deficient fatigue, the patient can reasonably rebound with some rest and/or food, but *yang* deficiency is described as total mental and physical exhaustion. Skilled clinicians will observe physical changes but also will hear patients express not having the "will" (in TCM this is associated with the Kidney energy referred to as, *zhi*, and yes, they will actually use the word "will") to continue allopathic treatment. We consider this a definite indication of serious decline, which the *Du* meridian can address. The *Du Mai*, especially in conjunction with moxa can be very effective to replenish energy and inspire greater sense of resolve.

Physiological Indications of the Du Channel	
Excess wind signs in the form of neurological issues such as infantile seizures, Parkinson's disease, epilepsy, stroke, hemiplegia, Bell's palsy, etc.	High fevers and restlessness
Numbness, cold and stiffness in the body	Sexual dysfunction, including low libido, impotence, sterility, infertility and low motility of the egg or sperm
Amnesia	Issues with coordination, balance and gait
Severe back pain	Hemorrhoids
Incontinence	Throat *Bi* affecting language and difficulty articulating ideas
Stuttering	Loss of voice
Prolapse	

Physiological Indications from Professor Mark Frost		
Adrenal exhaustion	Inflammatory conditions such as eczema, asthma, and arthritis	Immunity and resistance to disease issues

Psychological indications of the *Du* channel from Ann Cecil-Sterman[187]	
Strong aversion to responsibility and commitment	Overly independent
Overachievement without happiness	Hyperactivity
Always searching for something better	Holding the view that one is separate from the world
Keeping the world out because it is seen as perverse	Attention Deficit Hyperactivity Disorder (ADHD)
Failure to initiate action	The tendency to follow and never to lead
Shyness and/or timidity	Fear of being alone
Overtly dependent or a tendency to be clingy	Failure to establish independence
Failure to establish boundaries or tendency to break them	A lack of motivation, animation and enthusiasm; this can reflect in the posture and gesturing of an individual

Psychological Indications from Professor Mark Frost	
Mental stagnation, lack of inspiration	Mental, emotional and spiritual exhaustion

The *Yin* and *Yang* of the *Wei* and *Qiao* Channels

Historically, the *Wei* and *Qiao* channels each have been discussed as a singular whole, although they are recognized as each having two distinct aspects, *yin* and *yang*.

Together, the *Wei* and *Qiao* extraordinary meridians regulate *yin* and *yang* as it relates to day-to-day structure and function, essentially, providing the energetic framework of the body.

---

187 Cecil-Sterman, 2012

Specifically, the *Wei* meridians regulate the communication of *qi* between the nutritive and protective levels, while the *Qiao* manage the *yin* and *yang* channels on the sides of the body.

While the *Wei* channel's primary focus is on the regulation of *yin* and *yang* in the exterior of the body, the *Qiao* manage the transmission of *yin* and *yang* from the exterior to much deeper parts of the body.[188] It is thought that the *Wei* meridians keep a history of physical, mental and emotional experiences.[189]

The *Yin Wei* channel

Opening Point: PC-6 (*nei guan*)
Coupled Point: SP-4 (*gong sun*)

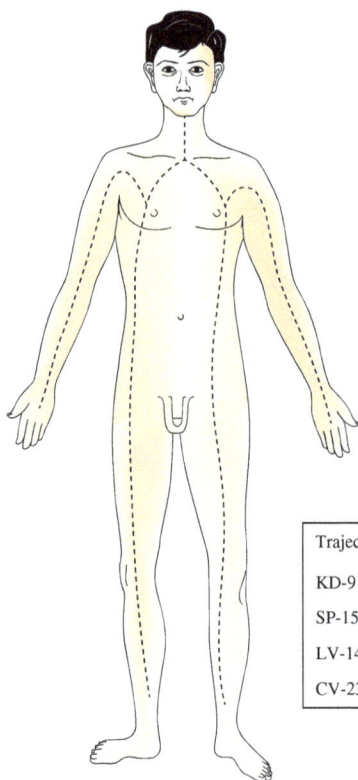

Trajectory Points:

KD-9 (*zhu bin*)	SP-13 (*fu she*)
SP-15 (*da heng*)	SP-16 (*fu ai*)
LV-14 (*qi men*)	CV-22 (*tian tu*)
CV-23 (*lian quan*), the channel then enters the brain	

---

[188] Chase et al., 2010
[189] Cecil-Sterman, 2012

Functions: Nourish *Yin*

Pathophysiology: The *Yin Wei's* ability to nourish *yin* is reflected in another translation for this extraordinary meridian: *Yin* Linking or *Yin* Gathering. *Yin Wei* nourishes *yin* through its ability to collect all the *yin* of the body and return it to the "Sea of *Yin*." Physical issues that present as a result of an abundance of *yang* or insufficiency of *yin* include headache and insomnia. It has great functional use in quieting and calming the nervous system to lessen anxiety, nervousness and balance hyperactive digestion that includes diarrhea, twitching, spasms, etc.

Yin Wei and Cancer: The *Yin Wei* treatment has become a staple in our clinical practice. The treatment is affectionately referred to as the "internal hug," and because one patient commented, "I feel like I just took an Ativan" it has also been termed the "Ativan treatment." Thus, it has become an indispensable component to clinical care because of its inherent ability to soothe and realign energy. Quite simply, when the *yin* of the body is sufficient, the whole person is grounded, nourished and calm. The low-grade anxiety that often accompanies a cancer experience is lessened by the foundation of the *yin*. The *Yin Wei* is also especially valuable during radiation therapy, a process that tends to burn the *yin* of the body and manifest with complex heat patterns both excess and deficient. Clinical experience indicates that this treatment is particularly effective in the first 2–3 weeks of radiation therapy. Each stage of conventional treatment causes varying degrees of anxiety, as patients understandably express worry and uncertainty. Thus, the duality of the *Yin Wei* to alleviate acute heat signs and simultaneously calm the spirit reflects its most extraordinary virtues.

Physiological Indications of the Yin Wei Meridian	
The five accumulations related to the *Zang* organs: Heart (hidden beam), Lung (panting), Liver (fatty deposits), Spleen (blood), Kidney (running piglet *qi*)	Men: hernia, UTI, prostatitis
Women: cysts, fibroids, tumors	Low back pain, which is heavy and achy and sometimes stiff and tight

(Continued)

(*Continued*)

Physiological Indications of the *Yin Wei* Meridian

Alzheimer's disease	Poor memory
Heart conditions: palpitations, arrhythmia, tachycardia, mitral valve prolapse, pain	Headaches related to blood deficiency

Physiological Indications from Professor Mark Frost

Patients withdrawing from opiates or anti-anxiety medications (the *Yin Wei* is the most powerful way to enhance the parasympathetic nervous system)	Gastrointestinal disorders such as ulcerative colitis, IBS, spasms, diarrhea, etc.	Migraines

Psychological Indications of the *Yin Wei* Meridian from Ann Cecil-Sterman[190]

Obsession with the past, desire for resolution of past disappointments, pain and trauma	Inability to accept the past resulting in shame and guilt	Feeling as though one is not in control of their own life
Emotional stagnation resulting in deficient blood from *qi* stasis	Sensing a lack of purpose	Pessimism, cynicism
Lack of motivation, will and/or enthusiasm	Visceral dryness and/ or agitation from the denial of the expression of the innate personality	Guilt

---

[190] Cecil-Sterman, 2012

(Continued)

Psychological Indications of the *Yin Wei* Meridian from Ann Cecil-Sterman[190]

Obsession, pensiveness resulting in stagnation	Asking "what if..." or wondering what life would be like if born in a different time or place	Resistance to aging
Anxiety about not being able to overcome the past, or life not turning out as expected or developing a hereditary disease	Suppression of memories	Throat *Bi* from an inability to talk about past trauma
Shen disturbance with blood deficiency	Nine Heart pains; emotional pain related to: finances, prosperity, career, vocation, health, relationships, adventure, children, creativity and sense of home	

Additional Psychological Indications from Professor Mark Frost

Feeling scattered, ungrounded, not in the present moment, not in one's body	Night terrors
Needing to enhance self-love, nourishment, satisfaction, completeness	Addictive behaviors

The *Yang Wei* channel

Opening Point: SJ-5 (*wai guan*)
Coupled Point: GB-41 (*zu lin qi*)

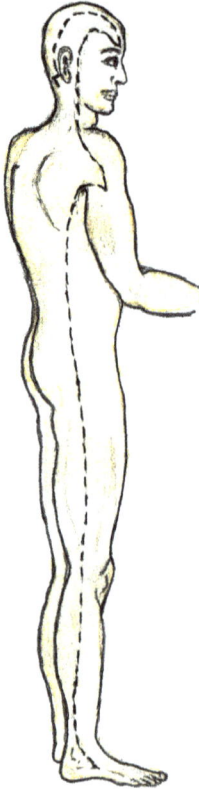

Trajectory Points:	
UB-63 (*jin men*)	GB-35 (*yang jiao*) (xi-cleft)
GB-29 (*ju liao*)	LI-14 (*bi nao*)
SJ-13 (*nao hui*)	SJ-15 (*tian liao*)
GB-21 (*jian jing*)	SI-10 (*nao shu*)
GB-20 (*feng chi*)	GV-16 (*feng fu*)
GV-15 (*ya men*)	GB-19 (*nao kong*)
GB-18 (*cheng ling*)	GB-17 (*zheng ying*)
GB-16 (*mu chuang*)	GB-15 (*tou lin qi*)
GB-14 (*yang bai*)	GB-13 (*ben shen*).[191]
Li Shi-Zhen left out GV-15 (*ya men*)	GV-16 (*feng fu*) most likely by mistake.[192]

Functions: The *Yin* and *Yang Wei* are said to rule the surface of the body. This makes for a wide application ranging from frequent colds and flus to a variety of skin issues. *Yang Wei* in particular supports the surface of the body due to its outward direction. Thus, it can be used to collect the *yang* and bring it to the surface of the body or the extremities. Because it

---

[191] Cecil-Sterman, 2012
[192] Chace et al., 2010

works with the surface of the body and is an extraordinary meridian, it is considered a last line of defense from deep, invading pathogens.

Pathophysiology: Whereas the *Yin Wei* is more about the inward self, *Yang Wei* encompasses one's connection, interaction and expression to the outside world. Its physical indications correspond with the immune system because of its close association with the protective (*wei*) *qi*. It should be noted frequent colds, flus, or compromised immunity that results in neutropenia are examples of conditions that may or should be treated with *Du* points, specifically DU-14 (*da zhui*). Similar to the *Yang Wei*, the *Du* channel treats skin issues and is relevant for cancer-related conditions that compromise the integrity of the skin. The channel traverses the spinal column and can therefore address muscular and joint problems, stiffness and pain. The *Du* meridian functions heavily in the physical and the building of *yang*. By comparison, the *Yang Wei* capabilities lie more in the mental-emotional realm to invite an outward expression of *yang* as needed, or restraining *yang* when it is too superficial.

Yang Wei and Cancer: The affinity for this channel to innervate along the surface of the body lends it to be uniquely appropriate for conditions related to the skin. From a preventative standpoint, the *Yang Wei* treatments facilitate healing of the more superficial layers of the body. Thus, its therapeutic range extends from minor dermatological irritations to skin cancers such as basal cell and melanoma. In addition to neoplasm, the *Yang Wei* addresses cancer-related symptoms that affect the skin and superficial tissue by guiding its healing efforts toward the injured area. For example, the cumulative effect of radiation therapy over an area of the body often leads to redness, itching, peeling and discomfort. The *Yang Wei* protects the skin throughout the course of conventional treatments to prevent further injury, while the acute presentation can be supplemented by traditional point combinations to enhance the therapeutic outcome. With regard to the mental-emotional elements of the channel, it is especially pertinent for the trauma of a cancer diagnosis. Patients experience an inordinate amount of shock, fear, denial and worry from the initial diagnosis and throughout treatment. Thus, the *Yang Wei* encourages the energy of the body to more completely acclimate to the rather sudden life change that coincides with the disease. This encompasses the entire realm of the journey, from denial to acceptance, which includes the possibility of death.

Physiological Indications		
Sudden fainting, stiffening, disorientation, dizziness, lack of clarity of thought	Lumbar swelling and pain	Chills and fever, wind signs and symptoms
Head wind conditions: Bell's Palsy, epilepsy, etc.	Low grade fevers, intermittent fevers	Chronic ear infections, chronic respiratory conditions, chronic sinew and skin conditions
Wei atrophy syndrome	Migraines	Herpes

Physiological Indications from Professor Mark Frost	
Various dermatological disorders such as: yin sores, non-healing ulcers, acne	Spontaneous sweating
Varicose veins	Bi pain in the extremities

Psychological Indications Included from Cecil-Sterman[193]	
Problems with decision-making	Lack of certainty
Post-Traumatic Stress Disorder	Being scattered, over-extended
A tendency to over-commit	Failure to prioritize
Difficulty managing a major life change	Difficulty socializing
Paralyzing fear, fright	Depression
Feelings of being empty and hollow, never being comfortable doing what one does, never being able to reach one's fullest potential	Failure to reach a sense of direction
Disappointment of not having achieved one's dreams	Inability to accept death

Psychological Indications from Professor Mark Frost	
Paranoia	Boundary issues
Outward behaviors, how a person expresses their truth to and engages with the world	Moving through time and transitioning through stages or challenging phases of life
Over-vulnerability	

---

[193] Cecil-Sterman, 2012

The *Yin* and *Yang Qiao* Meridians

Functions: The *Yin* and *Yang Qiao* meridians activate energy, both *yin qi* and *yang qi* throughout the body. Chapter 17 of the *Ling Shu* states, "It is simply impossible that there is a place not passed through by the *qi*."[194] Historically, the *Qiao* vessels were often viewed as one. In addition, the Chinese medicine concept of feminine *yin* and masculine *yang* influenced thought that the *Yin Qiao* has a greater predominance in women and for men, the *Yang Qiao*. This belief established a unique method of applying acupuncture points along the channel. For example, in a male patient, the opening point of the *Yang Qiao* is needled on the left side first. While *yin qi* and *yang qi* can be applied to different meridians and parts of the body, the *Qiao* vessels, being extraordinary meridians, gives them a sort of master control over the circulation throughout the body. This allows their use to be extrapolated in the possible roles of preventing cancer, or other diseases, by maintaining the *yin qi* and *yang qi* circulating throughout the body. This indirectly connects the interior and exterior of the body to address obstruction-type illnesses.

Pathophysiology: The path of the *Yin Qiao* channel travels along the medial aspect of the physical body; beginning at the malleolus, traveling up the inner leg, through the abdomen, chest and face, ending at acupuncture point UB-1 (*jing ming*). The course of the meridian indicates its therapeutic intent. The *Yin Qiao* treats the pelvic region for disorders related to the urogenital system, including the uterus and ovaries. Its range of action overlaps with the *Ren* channel both inherently *yin*-nourishing in treatment applications.

Its counterpart, the *Yang Qiao*, relates with the mechanism and nature of the *Du* meridian. Both inherently *yang* but each travel along different regions of the physical body. The course of the *Yang Qiao* reaches from the lateral malleolus, traverses the side of the leg, trunk, shoulder and terminates at the occiput. As such, it treats conditions that present in or relate to the posterior aspect of the legs, back, spinal column, cervical region, eyes and head.

The Qiao Channels and Cancer: Chapter 17 of the *Ling Shu* emphasizes the crucial role of the *Yin* and *Yang Qiao* meridians in the circulation of *yin qi*

---

[194] Unschuld, 2016

The *Yin Qiao* channel

Opening Point: Ki-6 (*zhao hai*)
Coupled Point: Lu-7 (*lie que*)

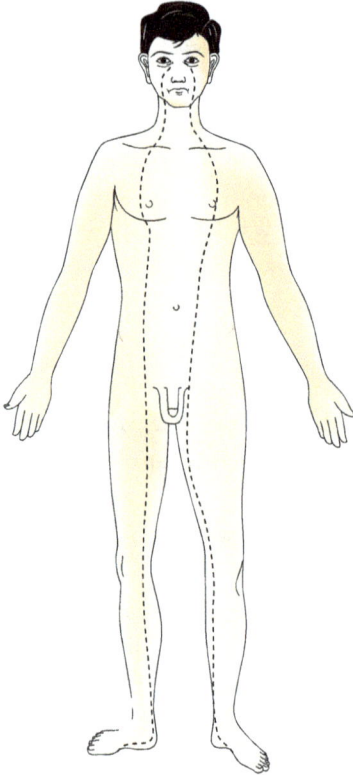

Trajectory Points:	
KD-6 (*zhao hai*)	KD-2 (*ran gu*)
KD-8 (*jiao xin*)	KD-11 (*heng gu*)
KD-12 (*da he*)	KD-13 (*qi xue*)
KD-14 (*si man*)	KD-15 (*zhong zhu*)
KD-16 (*huang shu*)	KD-17 (*shang qu*)
KD-18 (*shi guan*)	KD-19 (*yin du*)
KD-20 (*tong gu*)	KD-21 (*you men*)
KD-22 (*bu lang*)	KD-23 (*shen feng*)
KD-24 (*ling xu*)	KD-25 (*shen cang*)
KD-26 (*yu zhong*)	KD-27 (*shu fu*)
ST-12 (*que pen*)	ST-9 (*ren ying*)
ST-4 (*di cang*)	ST-3 (*ju liao*)
ST-1 (*cheng qi*)	UB-1 (*jing ming*)
GB-20 (*feng chi*)	

and *yang qi* in the body.[195] If the *qi* is not circulating smoothly, then knots or stagnations can form, which is a prerequisite for the manifestation of an obstruction-illness or potential tumor accumulation. Also, the organs must be in balance to prevent stagnation. The harmony of the organs and the circulation of the *yin* and *yang qi* have a reciprocal relationship for health. Chapter 17 elucidates the harm caused by invading pathogens that enter and lodge deep in the body disabling the free flow of *qi*, leading to accumulation. For example, if a pathogen lodges in one of the six *Fu* organs, the *yang qi* will abound and inhibit the circulation of *yin qi*. The insufficient

---

[195] ibid

The *Yang Qiao* channel

Opening Point: UB-62 (*shen mai*)
Coupled Point: SI-3 (*hou xi*)

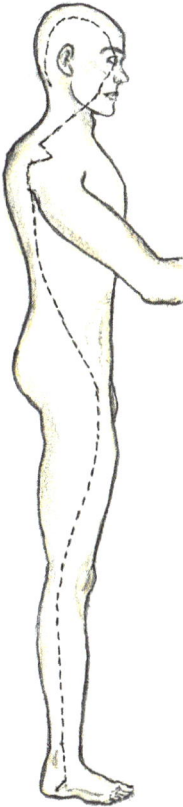

Trajectory Points:

UB-62 (*shen mai*)	UB-61 (*pu can*)
UB-59 (*fu yang*)	GB-29 (*ju liao*)
SI-10 (*nao shu*)	LI-15 (*jian yu*)
LI-16 (*ju gu*)	ST-4 (*di cang*)
ST-3 (*ju liao*)	ST-2 (*si bai*)
ST-1 (*cheng qi*)	UB-1 (*jing ming*)
GB-20 (*feng chi*)	

movement of the *yang qi* and *yin qi* disrupts normal function of the body and it is said that a person "…cannot exhaust their time of life and die."[196]

There are extensive ailments that correlate with neoplastic disease, both as a result of the pathology and conventional medicine. Among the varied conditions that result from the disease, cancer-related fatigue (CRF) weaves seamlessly throughout. The diagnostic pattern may indicate sufficient *qi*, blood, or *yang*, but the fatigue endures. Treatment with the *Yin Qiao* channel address the combined presentation of excess (stagnation) as a result of internal deficiency because

---

[196] Unschuld, 2016

of its ability to activate *qi* and connect the exterior and interior of the body. It is profoundly effective when combined with the *Yang Qiao* through the dynamic synergy of *yin* and *yang* aspect of the paired channels. In addition to CRF, emotional withdrawal and depression is exhibited with cancer patients, even those who tend to be optimistic and cheery. TCM oncology principles align this presentation with *shen* disturbance, perhaps due to blood deficiency that causes dysregulation of *qi* throughout the body. The *Qiao* channels are pivotal in shifting this type of emotional landscape through their remarkable ability to promote movement of the *yin* and *yang qi*.

The *Dai* channel

Opening Point: GB-41 (*zu lin qi*)
Coupled Point: SJ-5 (*wai guan*)

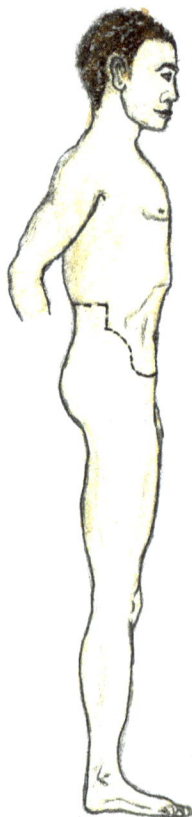

Trajectory Points:

LV-13 (*zhang men*)

GB-26 (*dai mai*)

GB-27 (*wu shu*)

GB-28 (*wei dao*)

Function: The *Dai* meridian is the only meridian among the regular or extraordinary with a horizontal trajectory. Its pathway traverses all meridians, and it is appropriately referred to as a girdling vessel indicative of its location that wraps around the center of the body through the abdominals and back. Therefore, its far-reaching influence acts as a boundary for the trajectory of all the channels and keeps the energy of the body unified. According to Chapter 11 of *Divine Pivot*, the *Dai Mai* has a connection with the primary channel of the Kidney through the divergent aspect of the Kidney channel.[197] This gives the *Dai* meridian a deep and powerful influence on physiological function. Li Shi-Zhen's inclusion of LV-13 (*zhang men*), the front-*mu* point of the Spleen, cements the *Dai*'s relationship with Spleen pathology as well.[198]

Pathophysiology: Classically, the two main pathological symptoms of the *Dai* meridian are internal abdominal fullness and discomfort in the low back that feels as though one is sitting in water.[199] Other conditions associated with the *Dai* channel are tenesmus, edema in the lower extremities, red and white vaginal discharge, menstrual irregularity, profuse uterine bleeding, seminal emission and protuberant type bulging. Physiologically, the *Dai* connects the upper and lower aspects of the body and regulates the upward-downward movement within. The *Dai* meridian is also the place where unresolved issues of the past are stored with psychological or emotional wounds. These are the deep-seated issues that affect and even determine core behavior.[200] It is thought that the *Dai* accumulates damp as a means to suppress these emotions and free the other extraordinary meridians from taking on the burden of these issues.[201]

Dai and Cancer: Unlike the *Chong* or *Yin Wei,* which we tend to use during certain stages of cancer, the *Dai* treatment is therapeutic almost any time. The energetic belt of the *Dai* meridian inherently harmonizes and regulates all the meridians thus affecting the entire body. The Kidney and Spleen's power arises from the *Dai* by virtue of their close connection. In the later stages of cancer, the *yang* of the Spleen and Kidney declines. There is a propensity for chills, internal cold, exhaustion, low appetite and general

---

[197] Rochat De La Vallee, 1997
[198] Chase., et al., 2010
[199] Frost, 2010
[200] ibid
[201] Cecil-Sterman, 2012

weakness. The classic TCM principle is tonify Spleen and Kidney *yang*, which can be accessed through regular meridian point combinations. Through the course of the *Dai* channel that acts as a vessel of collaborative energy, its range also treats depletion of the primary meridians. The outcome of extensive cancer treatment causes a myriad of injury to the body, but the incorporation of this eight-extra channel is applicable in early phases as a conduit of tonification, as well as late-stage with more prominent signs of decline.

An essential characteristic of this extraordinary channel is to lift, hold and raise the clear *yang qi*. This synergistically pairs with its capacity to promote the release of physical and emotional burdens. The psychology associated with the *Dai Mai* include: ruminating thoughts, overly controlling, not letting life unfold, obsessive overthinking, worry, anxiety or fear. These emotions go hand-in-hand with a cancer diagnosis given the immeasurable amount of uncertainty ahead. Clinical experience demonstrates the capacity of the *Dai* treatment to support the patient in such a way that they are more easily able to shift from denial to acceptance. As the most external of the extraordinary channels, it is an inherent link to the outside world. If difficulty or emotional trauma occurs and is not resolved in a therapeutic process appropriate to the patient, this energy accumulates and becomes stuck. A *Dai* treatment facilitates a release and emotional integration of difficult, stagnant emotions. Patients have remarked that with talk therapy they may intellectually learn or understand things, but the release or shift is more palpable after a *Dai* treatment. An important consideration is recognizing that the effect of any EEM treatment unfolds slowly, so there is rarely an immediate cathartic type of purge. The internal compass of the self gently aligns with the work in the days and weeks after the treatment. Although our present culture tends to desire immediate changes, this subtle approach tends to be easier and safer for the patient allowing for a more long-lasting change.

The scope of Chinese medicine is multidimensional, a synergistic system that has evolved through its own analysis of health and wellness. The versatility of the EEM illustrates this concept, and of the channels that encompass this unique classification, it is the *Dai* meridian that truly demonstrates this range in its ability to treat during any stage of cancer. From early, acute physical presentations to the physiological complexity of mid-stage and end-stage transitioning, the *Dai* directly benefits patients. In the specialty of TCM oncology, it is likely a practitioner will be met with questions about dying, or how a treatment can help confront the inevitability of death. Typically, patients express worry around the physical pain associated with dying or facing the mental-emotional and psycho-spiritual complexities of death. These queries arise as a natural response when all biomedical efforts have been exhausted. Mere observation of *shen* in the patient's eyes is quite telling, as the spark of the spirit begins to dim. This is a profound opportunity to remain present as a provider and to honor the patient's unique experience through compassionate care.

As true with all things, Chinese medicine, the treatment approach is dependent on the patient's presentation, but from an EEM standpoint the *Dai*, *Chong*, and *Yang Wei* must be considered for end of life transitions. The *Chong* has a connection with the Kidneys and Heart, which helps to connect one with their true self. Physically, it promotes blood circulation throughout the body, and thus is an effective remedy for pain as well as emotional connection. The inherent vitality of the *Yang Wei* channel encourages forward movement to accept the possibility of death. While these are equally potent treatments, it is the *Dai Mai* that we identify as the most uniquely suited for end-stage transitions. The *Dai* is interconnected with all the channels in the body empowering its systemic capacity. For example, it nourishes deficient Spleen *qi* and quells overthinking that accompanies this type of vacuity. The *Dai*'s correlation with the Kidneys addresses fear that is magnetized by weak Kidney *qi*. The acupuncture points that traverse the *Dai* are specific to the Gall Bladder and Liver channels, which move *qi* and blood in the body. Combine a *Dai* treatment with the appropriate TCM modalities, such as moxibustion or pricking techniques to achieve optimal integration with remarkable outcomes.

---

[202] Cecil-Sterman, 2012

Physiological and Psychological Indications of the *Dai* Meridian from Ann Cecil-Sterman[202]

Discharges: Leukorrhea, dysmenorrhea with white discharge, bloody discharge between periods, spermatorrhea, premature ejaculation	Pain during or after intercourse
Impotence	Urogenital disorders
Testicular pain	Prostatitis
Mucus or blood in the urine	Frequent urination
Mucus in the stools	Diarrhea
Edema	Sagging sensation in the waist
Inability to arch the back	Hemiplegia, paralysis of the legs, phlebitis
Infertility	Abdomen: cold-damp *Bi* obstruction in the abdomen with edema, bloating, cold or heaviness in the abdomen, obesity, borborygmus, intestinal issues with dampness

Psychological Indications of the *Dai* Meridian

Deeply-held trauma	Inability to let go of the past
Feeling unsupported	Resentment
Obsession	Stubbornness
Lack of spontaneity	

Psychological Indications from Professor Mark Frost

Lack of confidence	Repetition of self-destructive behavior(s)
Ruminating thoughts, obsessive over-thinking	Trying to control life and not letting it unfold
Unresolved issues from our past	

EEM and needling techniques

Classically, the eight extras were treated with relative simplicity: insert the needle, access the *qi*, leave it alone. Tonification or reducing techniques were not emphasized, but points were needled deeply to connect with the *essence* and to specifically address chronic, serious mental-emotional issues. There is debate among scholars of the EEM who argue that reducing or tonifying points is necessary to achieve results. However, we have found that due to the immeasurable cofactors that accompany the disease, the goals of treatment are reached with classical methods of needle insertion without specific stimulation. To interface with the *essence* of the person does not require manipulation, but just a mere introduction that allows the body to correspond with its own energy. As such, the *essence* of an individual is so precious that wrong technique or an aggressive stimulation will injure this vital substance, which cannot be repaired, unlike working with the *qi* that is relatively adaptable.

Other needling debates focus on the importance of needling opening points, and whether treatments should be bilateral or unilateral. Xu Feng, as mentioned is largely given credit for the development of the EEM opening points, but his fellow Ming Dynasty practitioner Li Shi-Zhen did not agree. He believed that the opening points were not necessary and advised needling along the path of the channel. Li Shi-Zhen was not a proponent of bilateral treatments either. Rather, it was only necessary to needle on one side of the body: the left side for men, the right side for women.

The dynamics of a modern clinical practice requires modification in technique and treatment approaches. So, while we agree with Li Shi-Zhen that it is not absolutely necessary to use opening points or needle bilaterally, there are instances when the opening point may not be accessible, or the area is contraindicated to needling as a result of radiation burns, lymphedema, swelling and pain. We have heard it said best by EEM scholar Mark Frost who likened using opening points or needling along the pathway to turning on lights. He further elucidates this by referring to a light switch; to turn on the lights, flip a switch by using the opening points, or screw in each light bulb by needling along the pathway. The synergy of opening points with those along the specific extraordinary meridian enhance the treatment effect. Those sequence of points guide the energy of the channel and integrate the deeper aspects of the treatment. That is not to say that the inclusion of other meridian points is contraindicated. Including points to modify a regular EEM treatment is therapeutically appropriate. For example, adding HT-7 (*shen men*) to potentiate the blood nourishing aspect of a *Chong* treatment, or clearing excess heat with LI-11 (*he gu*).

The duration of an EEM treatment parallels the flow of the *essence*, the vital substance that flows deeply and slowly through the body. The ideal time for any eight extra session is 35–60 minutes in order to allow this natural process to occur. Once the practitioner has determined which meridian to incorporate, points are inserted according to the classic trajectory of the points along the course of the channel.

In Summary

The Eight Extraordinary Meridians are a lesser-known method of treatment of traditional Chinese medicine in part because of various figures in history who have done away with or influenced large quantities of empirical evidence and understandings. The stories of their use being banned for hundreds of years in China are reflective of the respect that was held for this modality, and the understanding that they hold the potential to be a potent, life changing modality on the physical, mental-emotional and spiritual levels. While their indication for use in life threatening diseases is straightforward, their indication under chronic diseases may need to be clarified. Chronic disease in the case of the eight extra refers to those conditions which cannot, or have not, been successfully treated through regular means of treatment. With respect to cancer, it is precisely for the reason that the Eight Extraordinary Meridians have the ability to simultaneously treat multiple issues on the physical level and beyond, and their ability to treat when other methods have failed make them particularly suited for use with cancer patients.

Let us not forget traditional Chinese medicine was developed through a highly philosophical lens. Its concepts and methods have proven therapeutic for thousands of years by an untold number of practitioners. The EEM evolved within this paradigm as a system within a unified framework of meridian theory. This propelled an area of the practice to an esoteric realm the EEM reside in that is fortunately being rediscovered and synthesized by modern scholars and doctors of TCM. The ability of the EEM to access deep, physical and mental-emotional levels as they relate to cancer is multifaceted. The genetic influence of some neoplastic disease is scientifically known, evident in oncogene types and BRCA genes in women with breast cancer. Juxtapose this biomedical understanding with the principles of the EEM as interconnected seams of energy to the past (i.e. the physical and emotional traits that weave among families), then it is possible these meridians function to prevent disease imprints such as cancer or facilitate significant levels of healing.

EEM Highlights for Cancer

Eight Extraordinary Meridians	Cancer-Related Physical Symptoms and Signs	Cancer-Related Mental-Emotional Symptoms and Signs
Chong Mai • Tonifies Blood • Circulates blood throughout the body	• Headache, dizziness • Nausea, vomiting • Insomnia • Gynecological cancers • Urinary Dysfunction	• Connect with true self • Feeling stuck or unable to move forward • Poor self-perception • Panic attacks, anxiety
Ren Mai • Regulates *qi* and fluids • Nourishes *Yin*	• Gastrointestinal cancers • Abdominal masses (fibroids, cysts, tumors) • Respiratory issues • Difficulty swallowing • Dryness	• Issues related to bonding (excessive/lacking) • Propensity to feel victimized • Feeling incomplete • Neediness
Du Mai • Tonifies *Yang*	• Compromised immunity • Exhaustion • Urinary dysfunction • Numbness • Loss of voice • Adrenal fatigue	• Inability/lack of desire to move forward • Mental stagnation • Emotional and/or spiritual exhaustion • Timidity
Yin Wei Mai • Nourishes *Yin* • Clears Deficient Heat	• Heart pain, palpitations • Poor memory • Headaches d/t blood *xu* • Gastrointestinal disorders • Cysts, fibroids tumors	• Anxiety • Emotional pain from health • Inability to accept past • Emotional stagnation • Pessimism

(Continued)

(*Continued*)

Eight Extraordinary Meridians	Cancer-Related Physical Symptoms and Signs	Cancer-Related Mental-Emotional Symptoms and Signs
Yang Wei Mai	• Important line of defense against invading pathogens, disease (e.g. cancer) • Skin cancer • Radiation burns • Itchy, peeling skin	• Mental-emotional trauma • Dealing with life changes • Inability to accept the possibility of death • Challenging stages/ phases of life
Yin Qiao Mai	• Deep-seated fatigue • Neuropathy • Masses: urogenital, abdominal, breast, brain tumors	• Deep-seated fatigue • Withdrawn from the world
Yang Qiao Mai	• Neuropathy • Paralysis	• Rebellion or feeling powerless
Dai Mai	• Abdominal fullness • Inflammation • Edema in lower extremities • Diarrhea • Gynecological conditions • Frequent urination	• Psychological and emotional wounds, unresolved issues are stored • Release stuck emotional issues, experiences • End stage transitioning

References

Bella, G. D., Mascia, F., Gualano, L., & Bella, L. D. (2013). Melatonin Anticancer Effects: Review. Retrieved October 1, 2018, from https://www.ncbi.nlm.nih.gov/pmc/articles/PMC3587994/

Cecil-Sterman, A. (2012). *Advanced Acupuncture — A Clinical Manual* (First ed.). New York, New York: Classical Wellness Press.

Chace, C., & Shima, M. (2010). *An Exposition on the Eight Extraordinary Vessels.* Seattle, Washington: Eastland press.

Frajacomo, F. T., Garcia, W. D., Fernandes, C. R., Garcia, S. B., & Kannen, V. (2015). Pineal gland function is required for colon antipreneoplastic effects of physical exercise in rats. *Scandinavian Journal of Medicine & Science in Sports, 25*(5), 451–458. doi:10.1111/sms.12348

Frost, M. (2010). Eight Extraordinary Meridians. San Francisco, CA: American College of Traditional Chinese Medicine

Isabella III, N. (2004). The 8 Extraordinary Vessels — Lectures by Jeffrey Yuen. 3, 4. Swedish Institute.

Johns, R. (2009). *Acupuncture Techniques I*. Lecture presented at American College of Traditional Chinese Medicine, San Francisco.

Rochat De La Vallee, E., & Larre, C. (1997). *The Eight Extraordinary Meridians*. Monkey Press.

Twicken, D. (2013). *Eight Extraordinary Channels*. London and Philadelphia: Singing Dragon.

Unschuld, P. U. (1985). *Medicine in China: A History of Ideas*. Berkeley, California: University of California Press.

Unschuld, P. U. Trans (1986). *Nan-Ching, The Classic of Difficult Issues*. Berkeley: University of California Press.

Unschuld, P. U. (2016). *Huang Di Nei Jing Ling Shu — The Ancient Classic on Needle Therapy*. Oakland, CA: University of California Press.

Wang, S.-H., & Yang, S.-Z. (1997). *The Pulse Classic, A Translation of the Mai Jing*. Boulder: Blue Poppy Press.

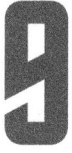

9 Therapeutic Exercise

"Strength does not come from physical capacity. It comes from an indomitable will."

Mahatma Gandhi

We met Lisa in our office two months following her diagnosis of stage II colorectal cancer. She recently moved to the area with her husband, who relocated for his job in sales. They were settling into the new town and routine when Lisa's digestive symptoms started becoming quite noticeable and bothersome. She complained to her husband about abdominal cramping and bloating. Then when dark blood in the stool showed up, this signaled an immediate call to her doctor. Just 36 years old, she shared with us at her first appointment, "I never thought I would have cancer. I'm too young!"

Despite the Western diagnosis, she was optimistic and determined to complete the conventional chemotherapy, surgical resection, heal and move on. After going through the standard Chinese medicine health history and intake, we asked if she had any questions. Her immediate question was, "How much can I exercise, what types are okay, and when can I start?" A devoted runner, she was compelled to maintain her routine and her body strength.

Lisa's initial TCM consult with us aligned with her first of six chemotherapy cycles. She had just completed her second infusion and while aware of the cumulative nature of cytotoxic therapy, she complained mainly of the acute nausea that affected her during the two days that followed. Her energy would rebound on the sixth day after an infusion, and she felt like "going for a light jog." One thing we have learned as TCM practitioners, and we are certain our colleagues and other healthcare practitioners would agree, it is likely impossible to tell a runner not to run despite injury or illness. Moreover, any individual profoundly dedicated with a particular sport or exercise will recoil at the very statement of reducing exercise to facilitate healing. This resistance combined with a cancer diagnosis lends to a rather tenuous conversation with patients, but one that is imperative in order to optimize their body's healing capacity and cultivate *qi*, not wipe it out.

The answer to Lisa's question leads us into this chapter as we explore the principle of exercise through contemporary Western frameworks, juxtaposed with the concept and function of exercise through the lens of Chinese medicine. To begin, both recognize the inherent benefits of physical movement in lieu of sedentary lifestyles to maintain sound health of the body and mind. While trends of the West indicate a hyper-focused attitude toward excessive fitness regimens to maintain weight and physique of the external self, Eastern practices emphasize moderation and the purpose of healthy movement to cultivate internal energy of the body, reflected in *Qigong* or *Tai Chi*.

Since we practice in the West, however, we must align philosophy with reality. This means we recognize that exercise has evolved away from daily natural movement as a mechanism for survival, to an activity that occurs by choice to manage levels of health and wellness. Movement we characterize today as "exercise" such as walking, running or weight-lifting occurred through daily tasks necessary for survival. This activity was akin to finding water, hunting for food, farming, building or maintaining a house. Now, exercise is a specific and separate part of our daily lives, and we have managed to further define it into different categories: aerobic, anaerobic, resistance, etc. The science behind exercise has also become central to an individual's purpose and focus, with emphasis on specific body parts, "such as the core" as well as cognitive training for the brain.

In general practice, we observe a theme among patients focused on body image, who are intent on losing a few pounds or more for a life event and are expecting an immediate return for their hard work-out and dietary restrictions. Therefore, their measurement of success is proven by the number on the scale. When results are not efficiently attained, they become profoundly frustrated, complaining that despite exercise and healthy dieting, "it is just taking too long" and they don't *see* a difference. While this sentiment should not be dismissed, we take this opportunity to shift the lens to the body's internal response highlighting the positive benefits happening at deeper cellular organ levels. Not to simplify the conversation, we reiterate gently, "Just because you cannot see a change in weight on the outside, there are phenomenal changes happening on the inside."

So, what are these benefits? It is well established that regular exercise improves sleep cycles that optimizes restorative functions of the liver and digestive system. This in turn regulates blood sugar, stabilizes metabolism and consequently assists in weight loss. The release of endorphins casually referred to as "happy hormones" also serves to regulate and improve mood after cardiovascular activity. These are vital components to maintaining longevity and certainly, cancer prevention. Proper execution of exercise for individuals with a cancer diagnosis reap great benefits and as integrative medicine physician Keith Block M.D. states in his book, *Life Over Cancer*, "...exercise may be crucial to your very survival. A sedentary lifestyle is a bad idea no matter what your health but is a really bad idea for cancer patients."[203] He cautions that inactivity leads to weakening muscles, a cause and effect process whereby malignant cells release inflammatory biochemicals that further degrade muscle tissue. An integral component to a healthy skeletal muscular system is the function of muscles to serve as a foundation for key proteins released from organs, ultimately potentiating the capacity of the immune system to encourage the good fight against cancer. Moreover, exercise increases natural killer (NK) cells that improve the immune system, as well as boosting macrophages, which are anti-cancer compounds within immune cells. The antioxidant defense system that protects against free radical damage also is enhanced by regular, moderate exercise.[204]

Given this brief scientific framework on the power of exercise for physical wellness, there is equal value in the mental-emotional relief achieved through activities such as yoga, barre, Pilates or even endurance training and cardio. Patients frequently describe the need to exercise as a means to "manage stress," and when they do not or cannot exercise, they report mental *and* physical disappointment. Patients have demonstrated time and again a visceral urgency to work-out to decrease stress sometimes

---

203 Block, 155
204 Antioxidants and Free Radicals, 1996

disregarding illness or injury. Clinical observations conclude this likely contributes to the addiction-like behavior displayed when it comes to exercise. Layer the societal pressure to appear healthy and fit with feel-good hormones and it is not surprising that the global health club industry generated over 83 billion dollars in 2016.[205] Nor is it surprising the health and wellness industry, as a whole, is projected to be the next trillion-dollar industry.[206]

A direct result of this trend is quite positive, however, as it eludes to a collective awareness that exercise positively influences the physical and emotional terrain. Through this scope of understanding, we bridge the gap between East and West exercise philosophy. This physical, emotional connection is a profound link within the modality of exercise because it harkens back to the core principles of TCM, which recognizes the individual constitution, its structural and energetic anatomy that never separates mind, body and spirit. Exercise is a prime illustration of the reciprocal effects each aspect of one's self has on the other.

Thus, the modern practitioner of Chinese medicine utilizes these essential concepts to determine the optimal exercises that align with a cancer patient's historical and current health pattern. Let's return to our young patient Lisa with colorectal cancer. She presented with a history of moderately good health with no past history of serious illness or chronic conditions. She was physically active and engaged in a variety of mind-body oriented practices. She attributed the acute gastrointestinal symptoms to potential food triggers or stress, reflecting that stomach upset sometimes occurred with emotional challenges. Despite the intermittent episodes, she reported that her digestion would quickly regulate and never affected quality of life to a significant degree, but she tended towards gastrointestinal symptoms. From the Western medical standpoint, there was no indication or cause for her cancer including no family history. By comparison, the Chinese medicine pattern identified these long-standing digestive imbalances as disharmony of the Liver and Spleen with concurrent blood deficiency. Untreated, this imbalance can generate stagnation of the Liver, depleting the Spleen and Stomach's ability to transform and transport food and fluids, which over time cause damp accumulations that eventually lead to heat and

---

[205] Statista, 2018
[206] Krom, 2016

toxicity in the Large Intestine channels or within the *Zang-Fu* organ system. Fortunately, we integrated Chinese medicine treatments at a point when Lisa was not overwhelmingly fatigued by conventional medicine. This not only allowed us to establish a primary TCM diagnosis, but it was a window of opportunity to utilize the modalities of Chinese medicine to optimize the immune system, regulate sleep and digestion, improve energy, as well as to answer questions and discuss supportive self-care activities, such as exercise. We established a baseline of health quite early that served as a measurement of progress and allowed us to monitor therapeutic changes. It is not always the case that we are able to collaborate care before surgery, chemotherapy or radiation cycles, as some individuals seek complementary medicine towards the end of Western treatments when they are profoundly depleted, creating significant clinical challenges.

One of the easiest methods we employ to effectively integrate care is to review pre-chemo labs for patients going through cyclical chemotherapy regimens. This is an invaluable tool TCM practitioners may rely upon to indicate optimal integrative therapy. It also sheds light on the matrix of the body, and its response to conventional medicine as a separate and objective interpretation. The lab values we review first are the neutrophils, which include immune system cells such as leukocytes or white blood cells. Chemotherapy can cause a condition called neutropenia, which signals a suppressed immune system and susceptibility to infection. As healthcare practitioners know, lab values do not always correlate to patient complaints or symptoms. So, we consider this another opportunity to utilize modern medical advancements and review the numbers. Further, precise lab numbers can fall anywhere along the normal range; even if it is low but within the parameters, chemotherapy is scheduled. Ask your patients for their pre-chemo labs. It enables more refined TCM treatments that improve the therapeutic outcome.

This was the usual routine with Lisa week after week. Just before her fourth cycle, her neutrophil level was low, and chemotherapy was postponed, which we always consider an early red flag of internal distress. The cumulative nature of chemo tends to rear its ugly head midway through prescribed cycles in a rather aggressive manner. While we attempted to prepare her body for this likelihood, Lisa's fatigue increased, nausea and bloating persisted, and emotionally, she was discouraged and mildly depressed with no desire to engage with friends. The prior success found in moderating acute side-effects while also maintaining normal levels of white and red blood cells with weekly acupuncture and moxibustion sessions had come to an abrupt halt. She reported low appetite, and so, we honed in on an updated nutrition plan, but she still only ate minimal amounts, which we assumed was a result of low-grade nausea.

As expected, a week off chemotherapy revitalized her sense of energy, which she reported happily. We delved a bit further into her daily life and learned she was frustrated with the "chemo bloat" and perceived weight gain. This was a clinical "aha" moment. We learned she was motivated by this "weight gain" to start "running the hill" next to her house, which essentially meant running up a long, steep hill and then walking up and down when she could no longer run. She reasoned that more energy indicated she should start exercising again, and "she wanted to take advantage of her energy" while she had it. We discovered this clear pattern occurred every other week always prior to a decline in pre-chemo labs. Postponement weeks are not positive reprieves or reward for good behavior. The time must be used to rebuild in order to return for infusion therapy as scheduled. Further delays compromise the efficacy of chemotherapy and can significantly impact tumor regression and outcomes. Consequently, we encouraged Lisa to focus on sleep hygiene, gently walking for less than 30 minutes a day, drinking bone broth, eating congee, continuing acupuncture and of course, doing moxibustion heat therapy at home as instructed. As a result, levels increased by the following week, and she was back on track with cycles. After the acute chemo symptoms resolved, we discovered she was back to running up the hill daily. Like clockwork, the following week white blood cells would drop along with her energy, and she would miss another chemotherapy dosage.

This is akin to filling a cup with a hole in it. We sometimes refer to this questionable decision-making by patients as "disease delirium." Chinese medicine explains it as the yang qi not rising to the head causing unclear thinking. After three rounds of this behavior, she finally understood her body needed the strength and vitality to recover. Another impetus to adhere to the treatment plan was to remind her that skipping chemotherapy was merely a postponement akin to jury duty; you are going to have to go back eventually. Moreover, continuing to exercise with that intensity was not productive, and in fact, it carried the risk of making her ineligible to receive chemotherapy *at all*, which would inevitably cause tumor proliferation. Ultimately, Lisa completed her chemotherapy cycles and is in remission to this day, likely running up a hill somewhere.

Lisa's story demonstrates that the desire to exercise is profoundly significant. This desire coupled with the belief that one is healthy enough to do so can be even more motivating. However, it is crucial that the exercise is appropriate to the person's current health and constitution. Quite simply, Lisa's exercise routine was not ideal for her fragile state. This was an opportune time to remind her of Chinese medicine's concept of balance to achieve health. During cancer, TCM modalities serve as a conduit to harness the power of the body to heal itself by building its internal capacity, and it does so beautifully in conjunction with conventional medicine. In this case, the patient responded to acupuncture, moxibustion, nutritional therapy and as a result, noticed an energetic rebound. However, she deposited that energy into daily runs, burning it away instead of letting her body use that energy to rebuild.

One of the interesting elements to this case was the opportunity to examine Western medicine's view on exercise during the treatment of cancer. Historically, doctors have advised patients against exercise and alternatively advised them to rest and let their body recover after treatment. In *Life Over Cancer*, Dr. Block notes this reflecting, "I recall vividly during medical training in the 1970s being taught that cancer patients should rest and reduce their physical activity after treatment." Recent analysis of how programs define and recommend exercise indicated not much has changed. We have heard this in clinic on countless occasions from patients, "My doctor told me to rest. I don't need to exercise during chemo cycles." This mindset is reflected in the American Cancer Society's (ACS) website that historically recommends exercise as a means of contributing to the prevention of certain cancers but *not* as a part of standard care during treatment. Recently, they have updated their website to acknowledge the benefits of exercise during standard care treatments, but it is long on cautions and short on specifics. The sluggishness and ambiguity of ACS is somewhat baffling from a Western scientific view because we know from a plethora of studies that exercise has inherent value to overall health, and with respect to cancer, moderate exercise boosts immunity and reduces cancer-related fatigue both crucial components to self-care during treatment. The good news for cancer patients is that this is starting to change, but the parameters of therapeutic, moderate exercise currently remain unclear. While oncologists or conventional cancer specialists recognize that cancer patients should engage in some form of activity, there are casual recommendations that do not entirely consider the patient's constitutional health, diagnosis and treatment outcomes.

For example, a recent patient diagnosed with invasive lobular breast cancer began Chinese medicine treatments to support her body before and during five weeks of radiation therapy, following lymph node excision and mastectomy of the left breast. The 46-year-old mother of two boys is physically fit and exercises at least five days a week, choosing among running, barre and hikes. She falls into the category of patients who say, "I *need* to exercise for my sanity." Chinese medical diagnosis correlates breast tumors with stagnation of the Liver, and the cumulative nature of stress that causes accumulations along the channel pathway, which for women is the breast. Thus, this patient's diagnosis aligns with patterns of chronic, untreated Liver *qi* stagnation with underlying Liver/Kidney *yin* deficiency and blood vacuity. During our consultation, she explained that her radiation oncologist encouraged her to continue her exercise routine and only prohibited swimming. She was instructed to just be careful of skin irritation and exposure to excess deodorants or irritants, which is the usual cautions with radiation therapy.

Based on her TCM pattern, we disagreed. Her body was already demonstrating systemic deficiency associated with constitutional elements and post-surgical depletion. In addition, there was the cancer itself, which requires vitality and stamina to fight the virulent, invading pathogen. Continuing to maintain her regular exercise routine would further compromise her energy and healing ability. The science around excessive exercise indicates that it increases oxidative stress and inflammation and can damage soft tissue, which potentiates cellular malignant spread.[207] We share this case as a mere example of the inconsistent messages relayed between patients and conventional medical providers, who certainly have the patient's best

---

[207] Pingitore, 2015

health outcomes in mind but are lacking in perspectives that consider the whole person.

Of the programs we analyzed, we found Dr. Block's "Physical Care Plan" as part of his integrative oncology clinic well-structured, taking into account physiological, biological and individual characteristics through mindful collaboration among providers and patients. This illustrates the core concepts of Chinese medicine that impress the value and necessity of creating treatment plans according to a person's unique constitution.

The studies on therapeutic exercise during cancer highlight another integral component of Chinese medicine. The principle of moderation. The term "moderate" is routinely referred to in Western healthcare, and this equates to the concept of "balance" in TCM. As illustrated in Lisa's case, her exercise was not moderate for her state of health, which caused depletion and postponement of chemotherapy. If it has not been stated enough, here it is again: a primary goal of using Chinese medicine modalities in conjunction with conventional oncology is to maintain chemotherapeutic or radiation schedules. This means it is of equal value to discuss exercise and physical activity with cancer patients in order to shed light on the value of physical fitness and health for cancer management with particular emphasis on the principle of moderation.

Extensive clinical experience has definitely afforded us an opportunity to reflect on the myriad conversations we've had with cancer patients about health including exercise. The dominant *yang*-like nature of physical fitness in the West is a cornerstone of overall health and wellness. So, the challenge is to weave TCM principles and approaches into the modern era with therapeutic finesse. The Chinese medical concept of exercise is what differentiates it from many modern-day recommendations for health or longevity. Specifically, TCM places greater emphasis on building one's internal health through gentle movement, exemplified in *Qigong* or *Tai Chi* practices, as a means to obtain overall physical health. These forms of movement essentially focus on the internal energy, then the external or working from the inside out.

This is in contrast to the relatively more aggressive focus of popular exercise methods such as high intensity interval training (HIIT), spinning, triathlons and body building that tend to cause depletion of vital substances, such as *qi* and blood by over exertion, as well as cause stagnation of these same substances through injury and inflammation. While there have been some cases of cancer patients insisting on keeping their membership to their local gym, most individuals recognize the limitations that present during cancer treatment. Just as it is a challenge to encourage exercise during conventional medicine treatments, it is equally difficult to dissuade patients from overt physical workouts, as illustrated by Lisa.

In either case, Chinese medicine values the meditative practice of *Qigong* or *Tai Chi* to harmonize energy of the physical body. Both forms enable a continuation of exercise, especially during active chemotherapy or radiation cycles when symptoms such as cancer-related fatigue, neuropathy, insomnia and other acute conditions present and inhibit comfortable exercise. The nature of *Qigong* and *Tai Chi* is to build one's energy and move that energy gently, which is not to say it is easy; it may even cause a light sweat! Patients have shared that daily *Qigong* movement, whether standing up or seated provides a sense of calm but also is invigorating. For mid- or late-stage cancers when the physical body is quite taxed, moving through the fundamental breathing and movements techniques of *Qigong* is invaluable.

There are many forms of *Qigong* and *Tai Chi*, but the commonality among them is an emphasis on one's breath. Life begins with the breath and must be nourished by it as well. These exercises build the capacity of the breath, harnessing *qi*, blood and in doing so, harmonize health. The pattern this process occurs through may seem quite esoteric for those uninitiated in Chinese medicine, and so, we will highlight the key concepts to create a foundation of understanding of *Qigong*. Let's begin with the Lungs, which are strengthened and regulated through normal respiration from a TCM and a Western viewpoint. A primary purpose of the Lungs in Chinese medicine is to govern *qi*, thereby influencing all physiological activity. From a five-phase/element viewpoint, the Lungs are part of the Metal element and control the Wood element, which corresponds to the Liver that is in charge of the smooth flow of *qi* throughout the body. Thus, the two-organ systems are interrelated and highly influenced by the actions of the other. *Qi* moves freely when the Liver is regulated and as a result the Lungs circulate air smoothly making it an ideal relationship.

When *qi* and blood flow uninhibited, stagnation cannot form, and any existing stagnations can be resolved. The air that flows into the Lungs is referred to as *qing qi* and is crucial to building internal *qi* and blood to supplement a person's *yuan qi* or primary *qi*, which ultimately supports Kidney *jing* or *essence*.

This delicate balance and free flow of energy and vital substances in the body influences the health of the organs and *jing*, essential for longevity and maintaining quality of life on a physical and mental-emotional level. *Qigong* focuses on this dynamic energy system to strengthen and build *qi*, emphasizing internal movement over physical exertion. Therefore, it is an ideal practice for cancer patients to integrate into their healthcare regimen during and after conventional treatment.

Now that we have reviewed the components of exercise from a Western and Eastern perspective, the following section will provide practical steps to integrating exercise therapy as it aligns with TCM principles. As true of all aspects of this medicine, professionals must modify as appropriate according to each individual constitution, diagnosis and treatment plan.

Diagnosis

With the modality of exercise, the physical fitness routines of a patient, whether they exercise regularly or hardly ever, influences TCM diagnosis and potential outcomes. Therefore, the pathway toward therapeutic exercise, from diagnosis to recovery and healing, aligns with the patient's physiological parameters at each stage. For our patient with stage II breast cancer, we explained to her the basic concepts of blood and *yin* in Chinese medicine and the value of these substances for vitality. Moderate exercise is encouraged, but her body's reserves would become further depleted by continuing an intense level of running during the five weeks of radiation and for at least one month after treatment. Therefore, we collaborated on an exercise plan that met her needs, both physically and emotionally, with an agreement that each week we would reassess and modify according to her body's response to radiation. This circles back to the merit and necessity of Chinese medicine diagnosis at each phase of care.

Inquiring

In diagnostic inquiry, asking is a fundamental component to a Chinese medicine intake. Every TCM questionnaire has a small section about exercise. While it may not seem relevant to a cancer patient's health history, it offers a great deal of information. Not just as a measurement of their fitness or cardiovascular health, but it offers insight into personality, energy, and their relationship with exercise. Do they like to engage in physical activity, or is it a chore? If they like it, what is their specific sport or activity of choice? How often do they exercise? How do they feel before, during and after? By comparison, do they practice meditation or *Qigong* to exercise their internal energy as well? Answers to these questions indicate underlying clues to their body's physiology as well as their mental connection and outlook to their physical health.

Making a Plan

Once the diagnosis is established and the questions have been asked, devise a therapeutically supportive exercise plan. There are several benefits to this approach. First, it requires the practitioner to communicate a diagnosis in simple terms for the patient's comprehension. This creates space for dialogue between practitioner and patient that emphasizes a patient-centered approach that empowers the individual. Second, it is an opportunity for the patient to reflect on their own exercise habits, whether nonexistent or excessive, and how their physical or emotional self responds to their preferred activities. This framework carves out the structure of an exercise approach that is adaptable to the stages of disease, conventional treatments and the patient's health.

To illustrate these three basic steps, refer to the chart below that provides an example of this process for the patient undergoing radiation therapy for stage II breast cancer. Each phase indicates a systematic process that assesses the patient's diagnosis, the role of exercise, and an agreed upon exercise plan that ultimately aligns with the patient's constitution. With each case, it is important to revisit this modality and make modifications as necessary.

Western Medical Diagnosis	Invasive Lobular Breast Cancer — Stage IIA	Radiation × 5 weeks
Chinese Oncology Diagnosis	Root: Kidney/Liver *yin* deficiency, Liver *qi* stagnation, Spleen *qi* deficiency and damp-phlegm	Branch: *Qi*, blood and phlegm stagnation in Lung and Pericardium channels
Current Exercise Routine	Active: running 30–45 minutes, barre, cardio + weights	5×/week
Modifications	Decrease: Running to max 10 min. of alternating 30 second sprints and 1 minute jog 3×/week Stationary bike as alternative.	Increase/Add: *Qigong*, full body stretching, range of motion exercises for chest, shoulders, upper back 3×/week max of cardio/resistance training for 30 min. 2×/week light walking for 30 min. 2 days off Stretching daily

Another helpful way for patients that do better with a more hands-on method is to take an "autoregulation" approach to their exercise and compare how they felt and performed each week with their latest lab values. If not familiar with autoregulation exercise, it essentially has the person adjust the load or intensity of the workout they are doing based on a comparison with how they felt and performed in their last exercise routine. For example, if a person struggled with technique towards the end of their workout and felt tired the rest of the day, then in their next workout they would want to lift less weights or do less cardio and compare how they performed and felt after. Usually, a patient will start to see a correlation between how well they workout and how they feel to their lab values. For instance, if a person saw a trend in leading up to their latest lab values of not performing well and/or feeling more tired after exercise and their lab values dropped, then this may be indicative that they are over-taxing their bodies during workout routines. In the end, this gives the patient something tangible to help them get the most out of exercising while lessening the risk of overdoing it.

Some patients will not tone down the intensity of exercise unless there is "science" behind it. If that's the case, refer to studies such as one in the *Journal of Endocrinological Investigation* that showed moderate to high intensity exercise, with a maximum oxygen uptake (VO2max) of 60% and 80% caused increases in circulating cortisol levels whereas low intensity exercise (40% VO2max) reduced circulating cortisol levels.[208] Too much cortisol for too long can have adverse effects on inflammation as well as other important aspects of health such as digestion and immunity.

A challenge in patient care is how to deliver advice in a way that meets the patient's needs in a manner that is clear. With this in mind, we try to summarize the important points in this chapter in the simplest language we can:

- It is important to exercise regularly during cancer treatment, but it should be done cautiously.
- Caution is advised because the ill-effects of standard care treatments are cumulative. The steroids involved and cumulative nature of the ill-effects makes it easy to overdo one's exercise regime. Overdoing it depletes the body and can cause delays in further treatment. Moderate exercise is the goal with the realization that what is moderate will fluctuate during the process of standard care.
- Regardless of one's exercise regimen, *Qigong* or *Tai Chi* should be included every day as its gentle methods have positive physical and mental benefits.

References

Antioxidants and Free radicals. (1996). Retrieved October, 30, from https://www.rice.edu/~jenky/sports/antiox.html

Health club industry global market size 2009–2016 | Statista. (2018). Retrieved August 12, 2018, from https://www.statista.com/statistics/275035/global-market-size-of-the-health-club-industry/

---

[208] Hill, 2008

Hill, E. E., Zack, E., Battaglini, C., Viru, M., Viru, A., & Hackney, A. C. (2008). Exercise and circulating cortisol levels: The intensity threshold effect. Retrieved September 12, 2018, from https://www.ncbi.nlm.nih.gov/pubmed/18787373

Krom, K. (2016). Health & Wellness is the Next Trillion Dollar Industry. Retrieved August 23, 2018, from http://www.womensmarketing.com/blog/2014/11/health-and-wellness-market/

Pingitore, A., Lima, G. P., Mastorci, F., Quinones, A., Iervasi, G., & Vassalle, C. (2015). Exercise and oxidative stress: potential effects of antioxidant dietary strategies in sports. Retrieved October 2, 2018, from https://www.ncbi.nlm.nih.gov/pubmed/26059364

10 Case Studies

"The doctors most learned in theory are seldom the skilled practitioner."

Edme Pierre Beauchene

Each case study contains all the modalities used to support and enhance standard allopathic care to augment therapeutic outcomes and quality of life for the patient. We are going beyond relating a simple protocol from a given modality with the goal of improving treatment strategy for the practitioner and to increase understanding of the possibilities of what TCM encompasses for those unfamiliar.

Case Study 1

Moxibustion Therapy for Radiation Fibrosis Syndrome

Synopsis
Patient: 59-year-old male
Western Diagnosis: Stage II laryngeal cancer
Chief Complaint: Radiation fibrosis of the throat due to extensive radiation therapy; localized pain, difficulty swallowing and speaking
TCM Diagnosis: Upper *jiao* phlegm with toxic heat, *qi*-blood stagnation, Kidney-Liver *yin* deficient heat

Primary Treatment: Direct moxibustion with dispersion method
Secondary Treatment(s): Pricking therapy, electro-acupuncture
Outcome: Significant, measurable, decrease in fibrotic tissue. Decrease in localized pain and increased ease of swallowing and speaking.

Biomedical Background of Laryngeal Cancer

Laryngeal cancer is a type of head and neck cancer, which are less common than other neoplastic disease accounting for approximately 3% of cancers in the United States.[209] Malignant cells are identified in the soft tissue of the larynx, a part of the throat that resides at the base of the tongue and trachea. The anatomical structure of the larynx includes three parts. First, the supraglottis, the aspect above the vocal chords; the second is the glottis, where the vocal chords are located, and third is the subglottis that sits between the vocal chords and the trachea (windpipe). The larynx is responsible for the voice by way of the vocal chords that vibrate when air is directed at them. Squamous cells line the inside of the larynx where cancer develops.[210] Major risk factors for this type of cancer include excessive alcohol consumption and smoking. Acute physical symptoms of disease may begin with chronic sore throat, dysphagia and inability to swallow solid foods, ear pain, awareness of a lump in the throat and change in voice, such as hoarseness.[211]

The Western medical diagnosis is achieved through various tests to determine exact stage and location of cancer. After a complete health history and physical exam, the patient may be referred for a chest X-ray or Barium swallow, also referred to as an upper gastrointestinal series.[212] This test requires the patient to drink a liquid with barium to coat the esophagus and stomach before X-rays are taken. Abnormalities can also be discovered through laryngoscopy, in which a thin tube-like structure is inserted into the larynx to view and remove tissue samples. If this occurs the tissue is taken to pathology to screen for cancer. Other imaging may be required

---

[209] ASCO, 2017
[210] NIH, 2018
[211] ibid
[212] ibid

like computed tomography (CT scan), positron emission tomography (PET scan), and bone scan.[213]

The standard of care in conventional medicine for laryngeal cancer include the following: surgery, chemotherapy, radiation therapy. The method and course of treatment is dependent on multiple factors like degree of spread, type, stage and health of the individual. External beam radiation therapy (EBRT) is a common method of treating many types of cancer, including those of the head and neck.[214] A machine functions by creating small beams of electromagnetic waves (radiation) that permeate the tissue in precise locations to eradicate cellular disease. Prolonged radiation therapy can cause a host of side effects, from superficial erythema of the skin, and local sensitivity, to deeper and more progressive clinical symptoms in the fibers of muscle and soft tissue.[215]

The effects of radiation can result in a condition referred to as radiation fibrosis syndrome (RFS). The tissue in the surrounding area becomes fibrotic, hardening into a firm mass, which in the case of head and neck cancers, can impact the vocal chords, esophagus, and ability to eat, speak and breathe normally.[216] Once this occurs there are very limited treatment options. Physical therapy and speech rehabilitation is necessary in most cases. Massage, heat therapy or myofascial release is cautioned due to the conventional understanding that local manipulation or heat application would lead to internal irritation and inflammation.

TCM Background of Laryngeal Cancer

This patient was referred to our Chinese medicine clinic approximately 11 months after the Western medical procedures. A thorough intake indicated the RFS impacted activities of daily living and overall well-being. Three-month follow-ups with his oncologist confirmed he was cancer free. Despite being cleared of malignancy, the patient expressed immense frustration with the tracheostomy tube. According to the patient, "The doctors and

---

[213] NIH, 2018
[214] Ibid
[215] Ibid
[216] Hojan, 2014

therapists have nothing else to offer. They say I just have to wait it out and hope the fibrosis decreases."

With ease, he used his tracheostomy tube to describe his symptoms. Stating that internally his throat felt extremely dense. He was acutely aware of an immobile mass that never decreased in size. He gestured to his throat and pressed firmly along the sides of the throat, across the scalenes, bilaterally. As he pushed, he said it was "hard as a rock." There was no report of pain, but he explained that he could feel tenderness and swelling inside the throat locally. The extensive swollen area extended from just above the laryngeal prominence, to the jugular notch and approximately four inches lateral in both directions.

Palpation by both practitioners exhibited hardened, fibrotic tissue, warm to the touch, swollen, and visibly red. Applying pressure did not elicit pain. He explained there was a constant need to clear his throat, with a mild, chronic cough because of phlegm and sputum that would not flush naturally through his throat. He wore an ascot around his neck, which, at the time of the initial treatment, was adjusted to its largest circumference.

He continued to explain that the previous year had clearly affected his physical and emotional health. His energy and stamina were reported as very low, he required sleep medications to fall and stay asleep, and maintained a long history of insomnia. His body tended toward hot, with desire for cold drinks, and a constant dry mouth. Prior to his cancer diagnosis, he was treated for asthma, which required the use of inhalers during activity. His blood pressure was elevated requiring prescriptions. He experienced occasional headaches and reported digestion as normal. Prescription medication included Vicodin (as needed), Prozac, Lisinopril, Xanax.

Examination of the patient's tongue and pulse demonstrated a mixed syndrome. This is often true with individuals diagnosed with cancer and complex disease patterns. The tongue body was red with deep cracks in the middle-upper *jiaos*, and a greasy-yellow coat in the rear. The pulse furthered this pattern. The Liver was wiry-full, Spleen slippery, Kidneys deep, thin, and the overall rate was rapid.

TCM Diagnosis

Upper *jiao* phlegm with toxic heat, *qi*-blood stagnation, Kidney-Liver *yin* deficient heat

TCM Treatment Principle

Dissolve phlegm, clear toxic heat, move *qi* and blood, clear deficient heat, nourish *yin* and calm spirit.

Treatment #1

Tongue: Red, deep cracks, sticky yellow coat
Pulse: wiry, *chi* positions deep, Lung/Heart excess, slippery, slightly rapid

Acupuncture
- Open *Ren*: LU-7 (*lie que*), K-6 (*zhao hai*)
  - Pathway of the *Ren* channel courses through the throat
  - Combination of extraordinary meridians nourishes *yin*
- Open *Chong*: SP-4 (*gong sun*), PC-6 (*nei guan*)
- *Ren*-6 (*qi hai*), *Ren*-12 (*zhong wan*), *Ren*-14 (*ju que*), *Ren*-22 (*tian tu*)
  - Palpation along the *Ren* meridian exhibited skin changes in tone, texture, and temperature on the above noted points, which were then needled in dispersing method
- LV-14 (*qi men*)
  - Spread Liver *qi*
- ST-40 (*feng long*)
  - Clear Phlegm
- SP-9 (*yin ling quan*)
  - Clear Damp
- Local: 2 *ashi* points on each side of the throat, approximately on Large Intestine channel

Moxibustion: Dispersing technique, direct cones placed in 4 positions on throat and each applied three times. Please see Chapter 4 on moxa techniques for a detailed description of dispersing technique.

Immediately following this treatment, palpation on the throat and neck demonstrated soft, more malleable tissue, and it shifted slightly with pressure. When the patient was asked to swallow, he reported that the mass of rigid, fibrotic tissue that enveloped his throat had lessened, allowing more movement when he swallowed. The yellow coat on the tongue dispersed, his pulses slowed to a normal rate, and visually, the systemic redness and inflammation that was present on his cheeks, forehead, and overall skin tone, lessened.

Treatment #2

The patient returned two weeks later and reported he was able to decrease the length of his ascot size down to a smaller clasp. He was very encouraged by this quick response. Palpation indicated smaller mass circumference and the edges of the fibrotic area were less rigid. He noted improvement in his ability to swallow solid food, and a decrease in the tendency to clear his throat from rattling phlegm. He reported that he did not need to take Vicodin during this two-week period for throat pain. However, the patient disclosed a long history of alcoholism and stated he was beginning to attend sobriety meetings. Given that alcohol is a primary risk factor for laryngeal cancer, the cellular pathology is rooted in this condition, but it also illustrates deeper emotional roots and complex patterns that correlate to his overall well-being and health.

The subsequent treatment plan included moxibustion, auricular acupuncture to support alcohol withdrawal and an Eight Extraordinary Meridian (EEM) protocol utilizing the *Dai* meridian to dredge and open the Liver and Gallbladder, to clear heat, detoxify the system, move and regulate *qi*. The *Dai* treatment is indicated for emotional releasing and letting go, also therapeutically relevant for this patient.

Tongue: red, deep cracks, sticky yellow coat
Pulse: wiry, Kidney deep-thin, Lung/Heart slippery, slightly rapid

Acupuncture
- Auricular (bilateral): *Shen Men*, Liver, Lung 1 (*zhong fu*), Sympathetic, Kidney
- Open *Dai* GB-41 (*zu lin qi*) (left first), LV-13 (*zhang men*), GB-26 (*dai mai*), GB-28 (*wei dao*), Ren-15 (*jiu wei*)
- Throat (local needles), bilateral, needle angled medially toward the mass, inserted approximately ½ *cun*

- ○ Electrical stimulation (e-stim) leads were placed on four of the throat needles, 10 hz, increased slowly to a level where the patient reported a noticeable, continuous frequency
- Needles retained for 20 minutes
- *Zhen Gu Shui* was applied topically at the end of the session to the throat

Moxibustion: Indirect heat applied with smoky moxa over areas of significant hardness using the dispersing method. The moxa stick is held over the identified point, with the practitioner's hand placed between the heat and the skin to moderate temperature. The moxa is held until the heat escalates, and then the stick is pulled away for a moment before returning to the same position. The point is not covered with the supporting hand in order to disperse the heat.

Treatment #3

The patient returned to the clinic one week after the second session. The circumference of the mass had decreased in size significantly, which was confirmed by the patient noting the ascot size was now at its tightest possible placement. He reported that internally, his throat felt less inflamed, large, and swollen and had "opened up." There was also an evident shift in his emotional state, observable from both the practitioner's perspective but also shared by the patient and independently confirmed by his daughter. He was making decisions to return to rehab for his alcoholism and expressed more optimism about his health and the future.

Tongue: Red, deep cracks, thin yellow coat
Pulse: wiry, rapid; Lung/Heart thin, slippery

Acupuncture
- LI-4 (*he gu*), LV-3 (*tai chong*)
  - ○ Classic "4 Gates" point combination to circulate *qi*-blood, move the Liver, tonify *qi*

- ST-40 (*feng long*), SP-9 (*yin ling quan*)
  - Resolve Damp and Phlegm Accumulation
- *Ren*-17 (*dan zhong*), Ren-22 (*tian tu*)
  - Open the chest and throat, descend rebellious *qi*
- ST-25 (*tian shu*), Ren-12 (*zhong wan*), Ren-6 (*qi hai*)
  - Classic "4 Doors" point combination to regulate digestion, by nourishing Spleen-Stomach *qi*, tonify and raise *qi*
- Local *Ashi*: approximately six acupoints along the lateral aspect of the mass, bilaterally, according to palpation
- Electro-acupuncture attached on all six-point locations beginning with 10 Hz
- Pricking therapy at ST-45 (*li dui*), bilaterally
  - In-out needling method to clear heat
  - The Stomach channel descends from the orbital region, through the throat, culminating on the 2nd toe at ST-45 (*li dui*)

Moxibustion: Indirect, dispersion technique along the throat combined with four rounds of direct cones on two local areas where thicker fibrotic tissue remained.

After the third treatment, the patient called to report positive changes in the mass and associated symptoms but decided to return to a rehabilitation center to address his alcoholism. So, although the course of treatment is quite short and not the preferred duration to properly treat his concerns, both practitioners were optimistic that with ongoing treatments the fibrotic tissue would slowly continue to soften and symptoms would lessen as a result.

Outcome

This case study illustrates the range of traditional Chinese medicine techniques in the treatment of cancer-related conditions, such as RFS. The side-effects of radiation therapy can extend from the superficial erythema, to deeper levels of soft tissue changes, requiring specific and refined approaches. Although the practitioners were only afforded three treatments to address a well-established condition, the clinical outcome was evident. It's also important to note that with just a few moxibustion cones and needles, immediate results were attained. This speaks to the synergistic aspect of TCM modalities and how treatments need not be overly involved, especially when appropriate modalities are used together, as they were intended in classical Chinese medicine.

References

American Society of Clinical Oncology: Head and Neck Cancer Statistics 2017. Alexandria, Va. https://www.cancer.net/cancer-types/head-and-neck-cancer/statistics. Accessed March 27, 2018.

Hojan, K., & Milecki, P. (2014). Opportunities for rehabilitation of patients with radiation fibrosis syndrome. *Reports of Practical Oncology and Radiotherapy*, *19*(1), 1–6. http://doi.org/10.1016/j.rpor.2013.07.007.

National Institute of Health — National Cancer Society. Laryngeal Cancer Treatment (Adult). https://www.cancer.gov/types/head-and-neck/hp/adult/laryngeal-treatment-pdq. Accessed March 15, 2018.

Case Study 2

Traditional Chinese Medicine Treatment of Stage IV Non-Small Cell Lung Cancer

Synopsis

Patient: 60-year-old female

Western Diagnosis: Stage IV non-small cell lung cancer. Tumor located on spine from about C5 to T5.

Chief Complaint: Primarily for recovery from the laser knife surgery six months prior to remove the tumor from her spine. The surgery left her paralyzed from the waist down and highly limited use in her upper extremities.

TCM Diagnosis: Kidney *essence* deficiency, Spleen *yang* deficiency, *qi* and blood stagnation

Primary Treatment: Auricular therapy in conjunction with physical therapy

Secondary Treatments: Dietary changes based on TCM theory, *Sotai* stretching techniques

Outcome: The patient had made little to no progress, per the patient, in the six months of PT alone prior to TCM treatment. With the inclusion of auricular therapy and adjunctive modalities the patient was able to regain strength and mobility to walk, and even dance, independently. As a side note, it was observed that her physical recovery had a tremendously positive impact on her mental-emotional well-being. This is pointed out to underscore the TCM idea that the physical and mental-emotional cannot be separated.

Biomedical Background of Non-Small Cell Lung Cancer (NSCLC)

Lung cancer is one of the most common forms of cancer, and statistically with one of the lower survival rates.[217] Non-Small Cell Lung Cancer

---

[217] Survival, 2018

(NSCLC) is the most prevalent form of lung cancer accounting for approximately 80% of lung cancer diagnoses.[218] NSCLC actually has various sub-types depending on which type of lung cell the cancer begins in, but the general name of NSCLC is used because the sub-types have similar approaches to treatment. Options for treatment include the standard care approaches of chemotherapy, radiation, surgery, targeted drugs and immunotherapy.

The patient, a 60-year-old female former business executive with no significant biomedical history presented to her primary care physician for the treatment of intense shoulder pain which, after three months, no longer responded to over-the-counter pain relievers. Her pain was primarily in the upper right shoulder. Occasionally, after physical exertion such as lifting heavy objects, pain would radiate down the right arm. She described the pain as having an intensity of up to seven out of ten, accompanied by a feeling of tension in the back of the neck. When the pain was particularly bad, she felt as if she must change her position to alleviate the pain (e.g., from standing to sitting).

After approximately eight weeks, three rounds of X-rays, prescription pain relievers and physical therapy, the patient began to experience several brief incidents of compromised balance and weakness in her legs. Her primary referred her to a neurologist who ordered a CT scan, which revealed a tumor extending from the fifth cervical vertebra to the fifth thoracic vertebra. Two surgeries and radiation followed which resulted in the patient having paralysis in her torso and legs, inability to control her bowels, and with extreme weakness and immobility of her upper limbs. Ultimately, the patient was left with a diagnosis of stage IV non-small cell lung cancer (adenocarcinoma) and told to "get used to a wheelchair" because she will never walk again.

TCM Background of NSCLC

The following six months of oral chemotherapy along with occupational and physical therapy resulted in little to no improvement in the patient's

---

[218] Non-Small Cell Lung Cancer, 2018

condition. At this point, she sought out a practitioner of TCM to help assist in her recovery.

With this patient, Kidney *essence* deficiency is characterized by the findings of both significant Kidney *yin* deficiency and Kidney *yang* deficiencies with some of the more classic signs such as loss of hair. The *yin* deficiency aspect would be normal and typically attributable to her stage in life. The *yang* deficiency aspect is no doubt related to her late stage of cancer, and a reflection of the damage caused by her Western treatment along with the fight against the disease. Her Spleen *yang* deficiency, which also is a reflection of treatment and stage of cancer at that point, showed classic signs of bright white complexion, cold to the touch, clear urine despite lack of thirst and little fluid intake, sloppy bowel movements, as well as a deep, slow, thin and weak pulse that was barely perceptible. In addition, there was likely some degree of long-term blood stasis present that coincided with the formation of the tumor. This pattern was likely amplified by her surgery that left her paralyzed. Along with her accumulations, she showed classic severe blood stasis signs such as purple spots on her tongue and lips, bluish-purple skin, and sharp, stabbing pains.

TCM diagnosis: Kidney *essence* deficiency, Spleen *yang* deficiency, *qi* and blood stagnation
TCM treatment principle: Tonify Kidney essence, tonify Spleen *yang*, move *qi* and blood, and stop pain

Treatment

Two to three treatments were given a week over a three-month period with one week taken off from treatment. The patient's complex condition opened up the possibility for a variety of treatment options. In the end, it was decided that it was best to focus the treatments on mobility, sensory improvement, and overall health. Support for pain relief was secondary because the patient had the option for medication, but a few points were easily worked into the treatment to help minimize the necessary medication.

Before treatment specifics are covered, it is necessary to point out that needles were not used on this patient. Her skin was extremely sensitive, and she could not tolerate any type of needling. In fact, she could only tolerate the lightest of touch without extreme pain. The patient attributed this to a side effect of her medication, Tarceva. Her extremely weak condition likely did not help the situation. As an alternative, a "Pointer Pulse" handheld transcutaneous electrical nerve stimulation (TENS) and laser were used for stimulation. This model has a 10 hz maximum stimulation, but only the highest level tolerable by the patient was used. Each point was stimulated for a maximum of ten seconds each.

Auricular points were the primary points chosen for treatment along with *Tui Na* to the affected extremities to reduce the pain and stiffness from physical exercise. Great care was taken to avoid stimulation of major arteries as well as the lymphatic system. *Sotai* stretching also was used to help expand the range of motion.

Principles from TCM's food therapy were applied to the patient's diet. These were given extra emphasis because the patient's oncologist did not want the patient taking herbs while on her medications. Some of

Primary Auricular Points Used	
Pain Memory	Found on the antitragus in the area of the limbic system, which covers the side of the antitragus and extends to the top of the lobe below the antitragus. Tender points in this area can be found relating to vertebral column, elbow, shoulder, ankle joint, knee, wrist, heel and hip pain. Lower limb pain was usually the focus, and these points can be found at the top of the lobe below the antitragus.
Master Lower Limbs	Located on the Helix Root. For pain, swelling, neuropathies, etc.
Master Mesodermal Tissue	Found approximately on the Internal Helix on the area that overlies the antihelix inferior crus and triangular fossa. Affects musculoskeletal disorder treatments.

(Continued)

(Continued)

Primary Auricular Points Used	
Correspond-ing Body Area: Lower Limb	Both Chinese and French points were checked with the most reactive points treated. The Chinese area for the lower limb is located on the superior crus of the antihelix starting approximately level with or just above the tip of the triangular fossa, the hip, and extending up to points below the superior helix brim (heel, foot, toes). The French area for the primary lower limb points extends on and slightly off a line from the tip of the triangular fossa to points on the triangular fossa and below the superior helix brim.
Spinal Motor and Sensory Neurons	Found on the descending helix starting inferior to Darwin's Point and extending down to the postantitragal fossa (approximately where the lobe begins). The motor portion is on the posterior helix and the sensory portion is on the anterior helix.
Point Zero	Found on the Helix Root in a notch as it comes up from the Concha Ridge. Through peripheral nerve ganglia it controls visceral organs to give a balance of brain activity, hormones, and energy. Basically, this point helps bring the body towards a place of homeostatic balance.
Thalamus (subcortex)	Found at the base of the Concha Wall where it meets the floor of the Inferior Concha behind the Antitragus. One of the main points used for pain control in the ear.
Frontal Cortex	Located over an area of the central lobe. This point initiates motor action and relieves motor paralysis.
Cerebellum	Found on the inferior antihelix tail and in the same approximate area on the posterior lobe. These points affect motor coordination, relieves intentional tremors and helps equilibrium as well as depression.
Sciatic Nerve	Located on notch at midpoint of top surface of antihelix inferior crus. Lower limb paralysis.

(Continued)

	Primary Auricular Points Used
Chinese Spleen (Left only)	Found on peripheral Inferior Concha, below the Concha Ridge (below Liver point). In TCM the Spleen controls the muscles and limbs by extracting *Gu qi* from food to nourish the muscles. The Spleen also makes blood from the *essence* of food and is the root of post-heaven *qi*.
French Spleen (Left only)	Found on peripheral Inferior Concha, above the Concha Ridge (above the Liver point).
Chinese Liver	Located on or around the peripheral concha ridge and concha wall. In TCM, the Liver controls the tendons and ligaments and is therefore important to their health as well as being useful for strained muscles. The Liver also ensures the smooth flow of *qi*.
Parathyroid Gland	Located inferior to French thyroid point on concha wall (French thyroid point is located inferior to concha ridge on concha wall). Relieves muscle spasms and cramps.
Chinese Kidney	Found on superior concha approximately below the tip of the triangular fossa. In TCM, the Kidneys store *essence*, produce marrow that in turn generates the spinal cord, is transformed into bone marrow, and generates bones. The Kidneys also govern water, control the two lower orifices, which makes it relevant for treating incontinence and also houses will power (*zhi*).
French Kidney	Found approximately in the central to lower-central region of the internal helix that overlies the triangular fossa.
Adrenal Gland (Chinese and/or French)	Chinese location: On protrusion of inferior tragus. French location: On concha wall close to Chinese Kidney point. Releases hormones to help with stress and inflammation.

(Continued)

(Continued)

Primary Auricular Points Used	
Shen Men	Found slightly above and central to the curving tip of the Triangular Fossa, approximately level with the meeting point of the Inferior Crus of the Anti-Helix and the Internal Helix. This is one of the master points. It is often used to calm the mind and support all the other reflex points. It is also good for pain, inflammation, stress, anxiety, insomnia, and excessive sensitivity.
	Specifically for the patient, this point was typically used in one ear at the beginning of the treatment and the last point in the opposite ear at the end of the treatment.

Auricular Points Used for Treating Diarrhea	
Interferon Point (B)	This point is located in the supratragic notch. It is said to be the Master Point for the treatment of all forms of diarrhea and have an anti-inflammatory effect.[219]
Small Intestines	Found on the Superior Concha above the Internal Helix Root. Used for diarrhea and indigestion.
Large Intestines	Found on the Superior Concha in the central part of the narrow portion. Used for diarrhea and loose bowels.
Point Zero	Found on the Helix Root in a notch as it comes up from the Concha Ridge. Through peripheral nerve ganglia, it controls visceral organs to give a balance of brain activity, hormones and energy.
Shen Men	Found slightly above and central to the curving tip of the Triangular Fossa, approximately level with the meeting point of the Inferior Crus of the Anti-Helix and the Internal Helix. This is one of the master points. It is often used to calm the mind and support all the other reflex points. It is also good for pain, inflammation, stress, anxiety, insomnia, and excessive sensitivity.

---

[219] Strittmatter, 2011

(Continued)

Auricular Points Used for Treating Diarrhea	
Sympathetic	Found at the meeting point of the Internal Helix and the Inferior Crus of the Anti-Helix. This master point improves blood circulation and balances the activation of the sympathetic nervous system with parasympathetic sedation.
Chinese Spleen (Left ear only)	Found on peripheral Inferior Concha, below the Concha Ridge (below Liver point). In TCM the Spleen nourishes the muscles and is also used for gastro-intestinal disorders.
French Spleen (Left ear only)	Found on peripheral Inferior Concha, above the Concha Ridge (above the Liver point).
Chinese Kidney	Found on the Superior Concha roughly on the midline of the ear (below LM-16, above LM-0 and Stomach point). In TCM the Kidneys relate to the ears and hearing, hair on your head and bone among other relationships.
Omega 1	Found on the Superior Concha, medial to the small intestine point. It has an effect on vegetative stress, which includes digestive disorders and visceral pain.
Chinese Rectum	Found on the external surface of the Helix Root below the Intestines points. Diarrhea, fecal incontinence.
French Rectum	Found on the most medial aspect of the Superior Concha approximately where the Internal Helix and the Inferior Crus meet. Diarrhea, fecal incontinence.
Laser stimulation	Ren-8 (*shen que*) and Ren-6 (*qi hai*) for 1 minute. Ren-8 (*shen que*) was chosen for its use on stopping diarrhea. Ren-6 (*qi hai*) was used to tonify the *qi* and support the *yang*.

the simple dietary changes can be seen in the modification of including fresh ginger (*sheng jiang*), lemon juice and honey to her green tea (*lu cha*) in the morning. Both fresh ginger and green tea have been shown to have anti-cancer effects specific to non-small cell lung cancer.[219] Individually, fresh ginger warms the Spleen/Stomach, supports the *yang qi*, and its

---

[221] Hessien, 2012

warmth can aid in circulating blood. Also, fresh ginger is well-known for its benefits in helping inflammation. Green tea is famous for its antioxidant effects, and its cooling property can help balance the warmth of the ginger. Lemon juice was added to the tea for its astringent function to balance out some of the exterior releasing action of the ginger and help with the diarrhea. The sour taste also will help generate fluids and *yin*. The small amount of honey added to nourish the *yin* and moisten dryness. The sweet property of the honey also helps to stop pain and tonify deficiency.

The patient was advised she should eat meals that were easier to digest, such as soups, to help take stress off her Spleen and aid its recovery. She also was advised to thoroughly chew food to help the middle *jiao* transform and transport. The patient was asked to observe how her body felt and reacted to different tastes and flavors but not to go overboard with any particular taste. It is known from Chapter 56 of the *Ling Shu* there are precautions to take with the five tastes. Specifically, that the sour taste goes to the nerves and is cautioned in people who have chronic pain or a diseased Spleen.[220] Also, too much sweetness can cause weakness in the muscles and the pungent/acrid/spicy taste injures *yin* and scatters *qi*.

A non-traditional recommendation was for the patient to begin taking daily probiotics. The strategy behind the probiotics is that they would act to help tonify the Spleen, and they would help with digestion of food, its assimilation, her bloating and borborygmus. Also, since most of the good bacteria that help people stay healthy reside in the digestive system, the probiotics would help strengthen her immune system. Outside of these changes, it was recommended she follow the principle of balance and moderation with her diet. Some would disagree with this and advise that she completely cut out meat and/or sugars. Overall nutrition still needs to be kept in mind, but when applying balance and moderation, good health can generally be found and maintained.

Regarding the auricular points, these points act in such a way as to treat the related deficiency and/or excess condition of the body, whichever is needed. Even with needling, there are no traditional techniques to tonify

---

[220] Wu, 2004

or reduce such that are found in body acupuncture. This may be for the reason that auricular therapy is more of a nerve-based system compared to the more *qi*-based system of standard acupuncture. Thus, for this patient the Kidneys and Spleen are being tonified, the Liver is being smoothed, the tendons are being strengthened, *qi* and blood are moving and points are being employed to help stop pain, as referenced, from a biomedical and physiological standpoint. Other points, such as the Spinal Motor and Sensory Neuron points were used to treat the numbness and motor deficits resulting from the two surgeries and subsequent incapacitation. Initially, the treatments began with fewer points: *Shen Men*, Chinese Kidney, Chinese Spleen, Master Lower Limbs, corresponding body points, as well as Spinal Motor and Sensory Neuron points. It was quickly realized the patient was able to tolerate a more elaborate point prescription that utilized most of the points previously mentioned.

The *Sotai* techniques were blended well with the *Tui Na* techniques, which further helped to move *qi* and blood and increase the patient's range of motion.

Outcome

Ear acupuncture treatments had an immediate effect on the patient's motor recovery. Within one week of the treatments, the patient was able to leave the wheelchair and walk 50 feet using a walker. The patient practiced walking five days out of every seven to improve endurance. The patient added intervals on the treadmill and recumbent bike to improve flexibility in the knees and ankles as she progressed.

Within one month of beginning treatment, the patient left the wheelchair and moved to a basic walker. Three weeks after moving to the basic walker, the patient progressed to a rolling walker. The patient used the rolling walker for one month, and then, she moved to a cane for three weeks. The patient quickly discarded the cane and now walks without any assistive devices. She reports superficial numbness in her upper back near the surgical site together with on-and-off stiffness in the right calf. The patient received ear acupuncture treatments for three months, considers herself 95% recovered and recently reported the ability to dance.

What is significant about her treatments with TCM is not just that she was able to walk independently, eat better and sleep better, but also the impact these changes had on her mental-emotional health. In TCM, we know that the mental-emotional and physical cannot be separated; meaning, that one impacts the other. The fact that this patient has lived well beyond her initially "given" time frame is important, but just as important is the *quality of life* improvement she has had. Instead of being immobile and depressed, she is able to live independently and enjoy the time with her family.

Even though the patient is not free of cancer, she is enjoying life. This is not because of TCM, and it is not because of Western medicine. It is because the two medical traditions were able to fill in the gaps and support the deficiencies of the other so that a complete form of medicine for the patient was formed.

References

About Non-Small Cell Lung Cancer. (2018). Retrieved from https://www.cancer.org/cancer/non-small-cell-lung-cancer/about/what-is-non-small-cell-lung-cancer.html

Fitzcharles, A. (2011) *Japanese Techniques* [Lecture]. San Francisco, CA: The American College of Traditional Chinese Medicine Masters Program.

Hessien, M., El-Gendy, S., Donia, T., Sikkena, M.A. (2012). Growth inhibition of human non-small lung cancer cells h460 by green tea and ginger polyphenols [Abstract]. *Anti-Cancer Agents Medicinal Chemistry.* **12**(4): 383–390. Available at: http://www.ncbi.nlm.nih.gov/pubmed/22043989. Accessed January 2, 2012. PMID:22043989

Strittmatter, B. (2011). *Ear Acupuncture: A Precise Pocket Atlas Based on the Works of Nogier/Bahr.* New York: Thieme Stuttgart.

Survival: 5-year Relative Survival (Percent). (2018). Retrieved from https://gis.cdc.gov/Cancer/USCS/DataViz.html

Wu, J. N. (2004). Chapter 56 The Five Flavors. *Ling Shu* [Translation]. Honolulu, Hawaii: University of Hawaii Press, p. 188.

Case Study 3

Improving Quality of Life in a Stage IV Pancreatic Cancer Patient

The following is a reprint of a case study article we wrote for the peer-reviewed journal Medical Acupuncture in 2015. A special thank you goes to the publisher of the journal, Mary Ann Liebert, Inc. for permission to reprint the article.

Synopsis

Patient: 48-year-old male

Western Diagnosis: Stage IV pancreatic cancer

Chief Complaints: Upper right quadrant pain, support through standard allopathic care, mind-body support

TCM Diagnosis: Complex and varied with focus on Spleen and Kidney *yang* deficiency, damp-phlegm, extensive *qi* and blood stagnation

Primary Treatment: Pricking therapy

Secondary Treatment: *Dai Mai*

Outcome: At the time of the initial article publication, the patient was about a year and a half passed his estimated life expectancy. During treatment, the patient experienced immediate, prolonged and significant decrease on the NRS pain scale. His physical changes included a more upright posture and more color in his face. What the patient primarily thanked us for was an improved mental-emotional state. He was able to enjoy life and time with his wife more with this shift. We attribute much of that to the work with the *Dai Mai*, but his decrease in physical pain certainly played a role as well. Of course, this is in line with TCM philosophy of the physical and emotional not being separate. His wife echoed his statement with emphasis on the overall improvement in quality of life.

Biomedical Background on Pancreatic Cancer

The pathogenesis of pancreatic cancer is less understood than other cancers with current statistics showing the five-year survival rate for metastatic pancreatic cancer at 1% of all patients.[221] Although conventional medicine treats patients aggressively and provides palliative care, patients generally experience a relatively minor impact on the disease. The treatment approach with metastatic and/or late-stage pancreatic cancer is to slow progression, increase longevity and maintain quality of life. Stage IV is determined by degree of spread, which is identified in organs outside the pancreas. In this case, the patient had tumors in the liver, abdominal cavity and stomach identified through PET scans.

The 48-year-old male patient prior to his stage IV diagnosis of pancreatic cancer was in good health with no history of pre-cancerous cells or family history of cancer. The patient sought medical care due to overwhelming fatigue, severe night sweats, sudden weight loss (11 lbs.) and pain in his right upper quadrant (RUQ).

The patient was metastatic at the time of diagnosis; therefore, surgery was not an option. Chemotherapy treatments began in biweekly, eight-hour infusions for a total of 12 cycles. This regimen consisted of a port catheter with 5-Fluorouracil (5-FU) dosed evenly for 48 hours after an aggressive chemotherapy infusion known as FOLFIRINOX, which is a combination of four drugs: 5-FU, oxaliplatin, irinotecan and leucovorin. The most intense side-effects of nausea and vomiting typically occur 3–5 days after infusion on average.

TCM Background of Pancreatic Cancer

The TCM perspective on pancreatic cancer is related to the Spleen, which is inherent to the proper function and metabolism of the gastrointestinal system from a Western physiological viewpoint.[222] In TCM, the Spleen has a relationship with multiple meridians, and its function is inherent to the balance and harmony of *qi* and blood. Long-term Spleen deficiency

---

[221] ACS, 2014
[222] Lahans, 2007

can lead to blood depletion that in turn affects the Kidney functions of producing marrow, building muscle mass and increasing oxygenation of tissue. A deficient middle *jiao* will create opportunity for pathogens and stasis to inhabit, such as damp, phlegm and heat. Further accumulation of heat burns the *yin*, and/or causes phlegm and phlegm heat to develop. The combination of the above factors may create an environment of blood stasis, as a result of underlying blood deficiency (poor Spleen function). When this occurs in conjunction with existing phlegm heat, blood heat will manifest and toxins, such as cancerous tumors, may develop.[223]

TCM diagnosis: Complex and varied with focus on Spleen and Kidney *yang* deficiency, damp-phlegm, extensive *qi* and blood stagnation
TCM treatment principle: Tonify Spleen and Kidney *yang*, transform damp-phlegm, move *qi* and blood

Treatment

The patient had no experience with acupuncture but was advised by his oncologist to seek help to cope with side effects from the chemotherapy. There were no other concurrent treatments or therapies at the time of our initial consultation or noted during follow-ups.

A Chinese medicine diagnostic pattern is inherently complex in a cancer diagnosis with presentations that change throughout the course of cancer treatment. This patient's symptoms reflect deficiency of Spleen and Kidney *yang*, indicative of late stage cancer. These signs include depletion reflected in fatigue, dyspnea, spontaneous sweat, lower limb edema, ascites, abdominal masses, and diarrhea. The tongue is pale with a greasy coat and pulses are soft, weak, and/or slow. There is also widespread *qi* and blood stagnation based on the choppy aspect of the pulse, dusky hue to the tongue, as well as red sides that illustrate heat in the Liver channel.

The patient was given three months to live. He's been seen once a week for acupuncture since his diagnosis for the past 16 months. Treatments were scheduled either one day before chemotherapy to improve his body's ability to respond to the infusions, or three days after to support

---

[223] ibid

recovery. As the patient's condition progressed, it became necessary to alter his treatments according to changing symptoms as a result of aggressive chemotherapy cycles. We chose to apply even more refined techniques to further maintain a more comfortable level in quality of life and energy with the goal of completing conventional treatments.

One classic technique found to be very effective for pain relief and overall health was the pricking technique. The pricking technique is an "in-out" technique utilized to effectively remove stagnation, clear heat, open up a channel or local area and/or stop pain. It may or may not cause a few drops of blood to come out, which are wiped with a sterile cotton ball until the color changes. An ideal outcome is that some blood is expressed. It is important to note that blood does not always come out, whether because of internal cold, *yang* deficiency, or because the patient is dehydrated and is not necessarily needed for the technique to have some effect. While opinions vary, it is generally accepted that a drop of blood is taken until the color, frequency, and/or viscosity changes. This technique was utilized with a 14-gauge three-edge Goldenflower needle on the left Liver zone, which is located on the anterior leg, below the knee, bilaterally.

In applying this method of treatment, the therapeutic goal is often one of a more superficial aspect; the results of pricking technique will immediately decrease pain, resolve heat and soften the quality of the pain. This is what occurred on cumulative treatments with this patient. With one to two quick in-out insertions of the needle in the Liver zone, drops of dark, viscous blood were expressed. Within moments of this release, he reported a decrease in sharp pain over his right rib cage, and the temperature of his skin in that zone of his abdomen, which was hot to touch, became palpably cooler. This approach was incorporated at the end of his treatments to invigorate blood and resolve excess stagnation to further promote this new movement of *qi* and blood.

Subsequent treatments included local pricking technique on the right upper abdominal region and rib cage. Specific points in these zones showed areas of small spider nevi or dark veins, reflecting deep, internal blood stagnation. While there are many indications for this technique, the pricking was performed with the intent to move stagnation/blood, clear heat, and stop pain. The patient reported immediate relief from physical discomfort after these sessions with a reduction in pain from an average of 9 to 4 on the NRS scale, lasting up to three days. Although these results were clinically relevant, it was not until the addition of the EEM that the patient reported both an emotional release and a physical one.

In addition to the acupuncture method of pricking technique, the *Dai Mai*, one of the EEM, was chosen to address physical complaints of abdominal pain and to support the patient in releasing negative emotions resulting from his diagnosis. The treatment goal is to support an integration of these emotions and provide an opportunity for release in both a physical and emotional sense. The *Dai Mai*, being the most external of meridians and having a connection with the outside world, makes it very effective for the releasing of emotional blockages both old and new.

An example of EEM treatment used on the patient was, in this order and beginning on his left side, bilateral: GB-41 (*zu lin qi*), LV-13 (*zhang men*), GB-26 (*dai mai*), GB-28 (*wei dao*), LV-14 (*qi men*), and Ren-15 (*jiu wei*). The last two points, LV-14 (*qi men*) and Ren-15 (*jiu wei*), were incorporated to bring the treatment to the present space. Specifically, the *Dai* was opened to access the deeper healing associated with the *essence* and to release stagnated emotions caught in the *Dai Mai*, while LV-14 (*qi men*) and Ren-15 (*jiu wei*) focused the treatment on the then-present physical and emotional chief complaints.

Outcome

Given the patient's positive comfort level, both physically and emotionally, and the fact he's survived more than a year past his estimated longevity, this integrative approach to stage IV pancreatic cancer has achieved the goal of improving quality of life. To control constant right upper quadrant pain, he has been taking Vicodin (5mg/300mg) as needed. He reports a decrease in this prescription dosage from three Vicodin per day down to one since we began addressing his pain with the pricking technique in the Liver zone. This acupuncture technique has had a positive impact on the patient's physical comfort and quality of life to the point that he described the treatments as "...a miracle!" due to the ability to sleep deeply without night sweats and an increase in appetite with the digestive ability to eat full meals.

Likewise, the *Dai Mai* treatments relieved the patient's physical complaints down to a 2 on the NRS pain scale but also prompted a release and integration of issues on a mental-emotional and spiritual level without the excessive use of needles or modalities. At the end of the first 45-minute session, his pulses normalized and tongue changed dramatically, which is an unusual occurrence. Specifically, his tongue coat substantially reduced, the size became more normal, and the color returned to a soft pink. When the patient left the office, he was standing up straight, color had returned to his face, his eyes were clearer, he smiled and spoke with a stronger voice.

During a follow-up session, he reported feeling well enough to take a long walk with his wife and enjoy a level of quality time with her that they hadn't achieved since his diagnosis several months prior. In fact, the patient's wife commented, "He was transformed by the treatment." With the exception of the inevitable, slow increase of Liver tumor markers, the remaining lab values have remained steady, and he has been able to embrace his life.

References

American Cancer Society. (2014). *How is Pancreatic Cancer Staged and Treated?* Retrieved from (www.cancer.org/cancer/pancreaticcancer/detailedguide/pancreatic-cancer-treating-by-stage).

American Cancer Society. (2014). *What are Survival Rates for Pancreatic Cancer?* Retrieved from (www.cancer.org/cancer/pancreaticcancer/overviewguide/pancreatic-canceroverview-survival-rates).

Chace, C., & Shima, M. (2010). *An Exposition on the Eight Extraordinary Vessels.* Seattle, Washington: Eastland Press.

Lahans, T. (2007). *Integrating Conventional and Chinese Medicine in Cancer Care: A Clinical Guide* (pp. 229–251). Philadelphia, PA: Churchill Livingston Elsevier.

McCann, H. (2014). *Pricking the Vessels: Bloodletting Therapy in Chinese Medicine.* Philadelphia, PA: Singing Dragon.

Rochat De La Vallee, E., & Larre, C. (1997). *The Eight Extraordinary Meridians.* Monkey Press.

Twicken, D. (2013). *Eight Extraordinary Channels.* London and Philadelphia: Singing Dragon.

11 Bridging the Gap

"Knowing is not enough; we must apply. Willing is not enough; we must do."

Johann Wolfgang von Goethe

The meaning of *bridge the gap* refers to the action of connecting two parts toward a complete whole. It requires participation among the divided entities to contribute in the unification of previously separate and different concepts. The hope is that once built, the result is cohesive stability. The concept of IO is in the midst of this assembly, piecing together many disciplines to create a relied upon practice providers and patients trust. The guidelines currently framing the system of collaborative cancer care are clear: conventional medicine is primary, complementary medicine is adjunctive and dependent on scientific criteria that is evidence-informed or measurable. This is the fundamental basis for integrative medical paradigms.

The underlying disconnect makes it difficult for holistic, natural practices, such as Chinese medicine, to fully integrate. Fortunately, traditional Chinese medicine is upheld by thousands of years of empirical research and observation of the physiological disease process. Classical interpretations of disease can be adapted to modern ailments. This inherent flexibility enables the practice to function by itself or in partnership. Thus, Western medicine and Eastern medicine adhere to their own theories, diagnoses and protocols to promote health and ease suffering. Separate sides of the bridge with the same purpose and end goal attempting to meet in the integrative middle.

To that end, it is imperative the Chinese medicine profession participate more readily in the evolution of IO paradigms. After all, a central modality to the practice is acupuncture. So, we must be part of the conversation and most importantly the application. We argue it is imperative not to become mere technicians in Western-focused healthcare regimes, recognized only for acupuncture therapy as a singular pillar. It is apparent that in large part TCM practitioners are drawn to private practice, where they can embrace ownership of the clinical process. The environment nurtures creative ways to implement a holistic, traditional medicine for the modern patient. There are plentiful options that reflect both the scientific, as well as artistic, side of the medicine. For the most part, we contend that this is preferred within the profession. Very few of our colleagues are vying for hospital positions. Essentially, private practice offers a broader range of treatment combinations as well as delivery of them with fewer limitations. The entire scope is at our disposal. If one technique does not work, there is always more to choose from.

However, the allure of employment in Western facilities is burgeoning. From a personal perspective during the clinical internship at CTCA, there was an initial draw to practicing as part of an integrative team. These positions offer a unique experience and opportunity to interface with medical providers. Such pioneers are responsible for demonstrating how Chinese medicine works to conventional medicine departments and also to patients unfamiliar with the practice. In many aspects, they are the first impression of the medicine, which is an immense responsibility to uphold. The outcomes that result as this phase of integration transpires are pivotal in determining the future role of Chinese medicine in IO. Although obstacles exist and currently inhibit the full scope of the medicine, the hope is that we perform with exceptional standards and skills leaving no doubt as to the merits of the medicine. The caveat is we need to be able to execute the range of TCM modalities without barriers.

Before this precedence is further established, the profession must first become aware of this incongruence. We intend this book to elucidate the current landscape of IO and from which, inspire practitioners to advocate for Chinese medicine in literal and figural terms. Often, the comfort of private practice beckons recent graduates who proudly hang a shingle and set up shop, where they remain. This is not to say those who follow that path are not contributing. They most certainly are. The foundation of Chinese medicine rests upon these small, yet powerful clinics throughout the world, which are applying the modalities, sharing and building the reputation of this therapy. However, while this occurs, the momentum of integrative medicine models is rapidly advancing and doing so without input from TCM doctors despite acupuncture being central to these programs. As a result, the degree of integration is determined by those who create the parameters. This pattern can already be observed in the preceding analysis of IO centers.

Fortunately, a beneficial component within the cancer specialty is the fact that all those involved are working toward the same outcomes: cancer recovery, remission, survivorship and ultimately, cure. The difference is the angle of approach, and it is aligning these angles that is the challenge. The biomedical methodologies focus on eradication of the cancer, inhibiting growth and metastatic spread. At this point in medical science, these techniques are more effective than Chinese medicine, and we are certainly grateful for them. However, the toxicity of conventional treatments causes undue damage on the physical body. In an effort to cure the disease, the patient suffers from adverse side-effects, and in some cases, cannot withstand treatment and succumbs to death. The good news is medical advancements occur on a daily basis, and treatments are becoming less toxic, more refined while decreasing harm and maximizing the desired result.

Chinese medicine must accommodate this evolution. In doing so, we diminish injury to the patient, both physically and emotionally. This approach cohesively bonds the very best of biomedicine and complementary therapies to optimize the healing potential and empower the patient. We liken these therapies as interconnected spokes on a medical wheel, each extending from the hub of conventional oncology. This structure depends on balance and synergy.

Research suggests at least half of cancer patients will combine interventions during their cancer experience.[225] Concepts of integration are driven largely by patient demand, and we could not agree more. A small survey of licensed acupuncturists in Northern California reported that of the 366 respondents, 77% consult with cancer patients.[226] The likelihood these individuals have created their own integrative treatment strategy is high. In our practice, we find this to be inherently true. Whether they realize it or not, they have designed a collaborative care team, armed with

---

[225] Seely, 2012
[226] Abrams et al., 2018

a nutritionist, naturopathic doctor, physical therapist, Reiki master, yoga and meditation practice. It is rare to work with a cancer patient who has yet to consult other nonconventional providers.

Despite this trend, there is a reluctance to share these integrated therapy choices with Western oncologists. By contrast, they are quite comfortable disclosing this information in our office. Patients study their conventional medicine doctor's viewpoints closely. It is common to hear, "My oncologist seems open-minded, but I don't know that I'll ask about taking herbs during treatment." So, we become the keepers of the collaborative treatment approach. The responsibility to interface with doctors, or other holistic providers on behalf of our patient rests in our clinical lap. Without a concerted effort to work in partnership, the disconnect continues among cancer patients and *all* their doctors. If the ultimate goal is to optimize the healing process, improve quality of life and promote curative outcomes, communication is imperative. The question remains how can TCM physicians and Western medical doctors develop more collaborative partnerships?

Integrative Recommendations

Awareness is the first step to creating change. We have established the apparent imbalance of Chinese medicine, and its role in integrative oncology departments. This is not to say every facility that offers acupuncture is prohibiting moxibustion or herbal prescription, but these are certainly the exception and not the rule. There also are advocates, other than TCM doctors, within these centers who condone further expansion of programs. Private conversations with medical doctors and oncology nurses offered insight into the undercurrent of desired integration. This indicates the potential for a wider range of therapeutic interventions. Similar to the concept of *moderation* in Chinese medicine, which encourages balance through cumulative changes in routine to improve long-term health, the same can be applied to the standards of IO practices.

Becoming Fluent: The Language of Medicine

In extensive conversations with Chinese medicine colleagues, a number have expressed frustration at lack of clinical resources in TCM oncology. To an equal degree, practitioners also have limited knowledge of Western cancer terms, diagnoses and treatments. In defense of TCM doctors, specialty training is limited. There are few courses in the master level program that cover the management of cancer, much less the diagnoses and treatments involved. This is illustrated by 345 licensed acupuncturists who reported that 44% had 0–20 hours of training in oncology.[227] Interestingly, 68% provided treatment for 0–5 patients with cancer within the past month.[228] Even in this small selection of practitioners, it is evident that a substantial number treat patients with cancer despite minimal specialized training. It is important to note that the concept of specialty medicine is a contentious debate in our profession. TCM principle differentiation and pattern theory is adaptable to any disease regardless of biomedical specifics. As such, practitioners do not all agree that specialties are warranted since Chinese medicine restores balance through its own methodology. While this is true, the caveat is that without proficiency in Western oncological protocols, the therapeutic potential of Chinese medicine is vastly limited.

Just as the TCM profession lacks an oncology curriculum, Western medicine is entirely focused on the scientific and cellular mechanisms of the body, and it ignores the greater whole. Subjects that are less methodical and measured, such as nutritional health and diet, are vastly limited in medical schools. In the book, *Anti-Cancer, A New Way of Life* by Dr. David Servan-Schreiber illustrates this dilemma, explaining that nutrition is covered minimally in a variety of courses, such as biochemistry and epidemiology.[229] Further, his introduction to nutrition, acupuncture, meditation and herbs occurred at a traditional Tibetan medical school. The concept of strengthening the body to prevent disease was foreign, "…my Tibetan colleagues called on remedies to me that seemed perfectly esoteric and probably ineffective."[230] His experience abroad highlights an integral disharmony between medical disciplines, as he explored two different hospitals, one conventional and the other, Tibetan medicine. At the former, his interactions with colleagues were familiar. They referenced

[227] Abrams et al., 2018
[228] ibid
[229] Servan-Schreiber, 2009
[230] ibid

similar medical textbooks, and surgery, ultrasound and other procedures aligned with the Western discourse. "We spoke the same language and understood each other perfectly."[231]

Thus, cohesive integration begins with the language of medicine. Without the ability to interpret and translate terms, communication falters. So, while each field is capable of explaining its own tenets and methodology, there is an inherent barrier to collaborative understanding and agreed upon applications. This does not imply that Western doctors should be studying the classics and memorizing channels and treatment principles. Nor should Chinese medicine physicians over-analyze pathology reports and follow the intricate dosing amounts of chemotherapy. However, both disciplines will benefit from broadening their knowledge base and become multilingual in the field of integrative medicine.

This process offers immeasurable value for both sides. Chinese medicine will profoundly benefit from learning core oncology terms for two reasons. First, it provides fluidity in conversation with a cancer patient. If the TCM doctor can facilitate an oncology intake that reviews the Western diagnoses, treatments, and medications of their patient, they establish rapport and demonstrate expertise. This invokes more confidence, crucial to patient-centered care and empowerment. Second, if the opportunity to converse with an oncologist or radiation specialist presents, there is an ability to interface with proficiency and skill. This in turn establishes more credibility for the specialty of Chinese medical oncology, and the purpose of which therapies are integrated.

Comparatively, if biomedical doctors have a basic comprehension of Chinese medicine concepts and its modalities, then the scale of integration becomes more balanced. There is less lean toward solely approving acupuncture, while rejecting any semblance of Chinese herbal therapy. Instead of immediately cautioning patients because certain methods are unfamiliar, there is an opportunity to explore holistic approaches. Indeed, this is a challenge for the scientific community because it beckons their participation into an esoteric medicine not quickly understood or easily measured. But, in order for true collaborative cancer care to evolve, it is important to establish mutual respect and knowledge of multiple medical languages.

---

[231] Servan-Schreiber, 2009

Applying fluency for collaborative conversations

The lines of communication between medicinal therapies is met with certain challenges. At its most basic level, there are physicians whose dogmatic perceptions inhibit aspects of integration. This is apparent along both sides. Quite surprisingly, there are Chinese medicine practitioners opposed to the concept of integrative medicine. In our doctoral cohort, we recall one practitioner who refused to treat an individual if they had taken any form of Western medicine within the past six months. This included aspirin, antibiotics and prescription medication. Only until the patient had followed a very strict detox plan would they begin treatment. This degree of opposition is appalling, particularly as modern practitioners working in modern healthcare. Patients are seeking complementary and holistic medicine in an effort to bolster health with more natural remedies in order to avoid conventional treatments. We are doctors who must facilitate this momentum with our patients and embrace these opportunities, not avoid them.

To a degree, TCM doctors expect to have mixed interactions with Western medicine providers. The process of reaching out to discuss shared patients is loaded with uncertainty. Concern of dismissal, blatant disregard or just being clearly ignored are also reasons practitioners may pause before contacting an oncologist. We have created integrative treatment plans only to have the oncologist promptly caution the patient against anything not scientifically proven. We assume this corresponds to a lack of knowledge about Chinese medicine, or perhaps a reluctance to explore beyond conventional standards of care. In the survey previously referenced, when TCM practitioners were asked how often they initiate conversation with oncologists or other Western doctors, only 8% responded *always*.[232] By comparison, conventional doctors rarely initiated communication with Chinese practitioners. The respondents reported that only 2% of the time contact was first made by the Western physician.[233] Alas, these similar patterns highlight the lack of dialogue in the medical community despite each being central to the patient's care.

---

[232] Abrams et al, 2018
[233] ibid

However, just as there are risks, there are rewards. Certain cases that provided opportunity to speak directly with an oncologist have been positive. For example, a patient with stage IV ovarian cancer undergoing aggressive chemotherapy cycles asked if we would speak to her doctor about the recommended herbal prescription. The formula addressed the apparent depletion of her body. In TCM terms, this included Spleen and Kidney *yang* decline reflective of the stage and progression of the disease. Specific herbs were included to support her vital *qi* as well as calm her spirit. Understanding the Western diagnosis, chemotherapeutic regimen, prescription medications and the patient's concurrent conditions allowed the conversation to flow between Western practices and Chinese medicine principles and treatment approaches. Within a short time, the oncologist began asking more questions about acupuncture, Chinese herbs, and how the medicine worked alongside conventional methods. This conversation inspired more confidence in the *possibility* of integration that reflects mutual respect among disciplines.

Logistical barriers to communication are not as easily manipulated. Oncologists and cancer specialists are in constant demand, often juggling patient care with administrative and clinical details. IO facilities offering conventional and complementary medicine at the same location have an added advantage of establishing consistent communication patterns. This is evident through shared electronic health records and weekly meetings among multidisciplinary providers, which offered a platform to present patient updates. This privilege is limited, however, indicated by a systematic review that demonstrated only 41% of integrative programs offered services under one roof.[234]

For the rest, conventional hospitals collaborate with complementary therapists off-site through referral programs. As an example, we are contracted with a major hospital as outside providers and receive authorizations to treat cancer patients with acupuncture. Unfortunately, this referral process only includes the patient name and chief complaint (nausea due to chemotherapy, post-operative pain, etc.). Health records or communication from the treating physician do not accompany the request, which forces the patient to gather their health information to share at their first appointment. While we request patients to complete the appropriate forms and

---

[234] Seely, 2012

questionnaires before the treatment, this is not always performed. Patients are impaired by physical discomfort and the shear overwhelm of the cancer process. Further, there are vast differences among patients. There are those who are familiar with cancer terms and treatments and have asked their oncologist extensive questions, like Samantha from our introduction, who had compiled a binder of information. Or, there are patients who do not have all the details memorized and are in a state of shock or denial. Asking about the chemotherapeutic agents, pathology or prescription medication does not always yield an answer.

Thus, first appointments have the potential of being rather tedious in order to properly gather and download the patient's case. The benefit of an initial introduction and exchange of information among providers establishes a connection from which a collaborative relationship evolves more seamlessly. Through trial and error, we have devised an ideal formula to encourage dialogue between patients, their conventional physicians and complementary therapists. It is not foolproof as we continue to modify and adjust through improved methods of communication that align with patient needs and integrative cancer models. This is a practical starting point for Chinese medicine doctors to create structure as they broaden their scope in the management of cancer. In our practice, it is a visual aid and tool that can be easily shared with patients, as well as their oncologists to promote collaborative relationships. The working document is a living entity of sorts, a collaborative demonstration and agreement that is modified throughout the course of care.

We have found it inherently useful to juxtapose the core components of West and East to clearly delineate the treatment principle and therapeutic approach throughout the course of care. The sections of IO start with the biomedical diagnosis, followed by steps taken to confirm it (diagnostics and staging), and the conventional treatment plan (therapeutic intervention). Additional information such as side-effects, are they already undergoing treatment, as well as professional advice from other practitioners, is equally important. The components can be modified according to the practitioner's discretion, but we recommend the following:

- Cancer diagnosis
- Western Diagnostics: biopsy, hematology, histopathology, tumor markers, imaging, etc.

- Staging: prognosis, localized vs. metastases, acute, chronic, local vs. invasive, etc.
- Treatment: chemotherapy, radiation, curative vs. palliative, immunotherapy, prescriptions, etc.
- Cancer-related Conditions and Potential Side-Effects
- Concurrent Therapies and Professional Advice: naturopathy, dietary, homeopathy, mind-body, etc.
- Supplements and Other Remedies: vitamins, herbal medicine, etc.

Depending on the individual's constitution, stage of disease and a number of factors, the intake may be quite extensive or conversely, quite straightforward. We have experienced both degrees, spending hours in consultation and review with a patient, versus those who are matter of fact simply stating cancer diagnosis, conventional treatment and physical complaints. Either way, we recommend starting with Western oncology details, preferably before the initial appointment. When this occurs, the TCM practitioner is given more time to analyze and process the patient's diagnosis and current health. This affords opportunity to research cancer diagnoses, therapies, and define unfamiliar disease characteristics.

It is from this point, assessment through the diagnostic lens of Chinese medicine takes place. Inquiry, examination, palpation and observation are integral aspects to the complete intake. More importantly, however, is the ability to discern the underlying (root) condition, relative to the symptoms (branch). The characteristics of active cancer, both the disease and the conventional treatments, cause a maelstrom of symptomatology. In order to formulate any aspect of treatment, these factors must be clearly distinguished to generate an accurate treatment principle. Once defined, optimal therapeutic techniques and approaches can be applied.

The oncology terms and definitions provided below are basic starting points to broaden medical vocabulary and promote fluid conversation with patients and doctors. As the evolution of cancer and treatments develop, so does the language within it. However, these fundamental concepts are the foundation of oncological medicine and as such, necessary to know for any complementary provider in cancer management.

Fundamental cancer terminology for TCM physicians

Biopsy: Surgical procedure by means of excision, surgical/needle or resection. A small section of the tumor is removed for histology and pathology analysis. Procedures include a needle biopsy, also referred to as fine needle aspiration (FNA), where a tiny sample of the tumor is taken. Resection biopsy refers to a process by which a surgeon removes the whole tumor prior to diagnosis.

Histopathology: The cellular profile of the disease and the microscopic study of cells and tissue. A precise diagnosis is determined through microscopic examination of the cells. This includes the histologic grade that refers to the differentiation within the tumor to assess size and shape. The grade correlates to degrees of malignancy: low is graded 1, versus poor prognosis, grade 3.

Differentiation: Healthy cells physically change according to specialized tissues of the body is referred to as differentiation. Abnormal cells are generally undifferentiated, often a sign they have been in existence for longer duration. Well-differentiated cells are less mutated. More aggressive tumors are undifferentiated, also referred to as anaplastic.

Tumor Markers: Substances in the body that can be measured to indicate the presence of cancer. The tumor or the body produces the markers in response to cancer. The lab value can aid diagnosis and/or indicate how treatment is progressing. For example, CA 125 is a protein and type of tumor marker. This substance is found in greater concentrations in tumor cells, particularly those associated with ovarian cancer.

Staging and prognosis

TNM: A universal system of staging to describe the anatomic characteristics of the tumor.

T: extent of the primary tumor
N: lymph node presence or absence
M: distant metastasis presence or absence

Benign: This term is associated with more mild disease patterns.

Malignant: A tumor that is cancerous and may grow uncontrollably.

Localized: Also referred to as *in-situ* indicating a tumor is confined to a single site.

Metastases: The tumor has spread beyond the primary site. Secondary sites may be adjacent to or distant from the original tumor.

Prognosis: The expected outcome of the disease. Influenced by factors such as stage, age, location, cancer type, etc.

Remission: Period that follows treatment, confirmed by analyses that determine there is no evidence of the disease.

Relapse: Cancer returns after a period of remission.

Refractory: This is where the cancer is resistant to treatment, patient may never go into remission, possibly with stable or progressive diseases.

Curative treatment: Treatment to eradicate the cancer.

Palliative treatment: Therapies that focus on pain relief and symptom management.

External Radiotherapy: Process by which radioactivity occurs from a source outside the body.

Internal Radiotherapy: Radioactive implants are placed in the body in or near the tumor to kill the cancer cells. Also termed brachytherapy.

Chemotherapy: Type of cancer treatment that utilizes one or more cancer drugs to eradicate disease as part of standardized care.

Cytotoxic: The classification of chemotherapeutic agents is dependent on cytotoxicity. This refers to the chemical potency of medicinal drugs that destroy cancer cells by inhibiting growth or multiplying during phases of the cell's life cycle.

Nadir: This refers to a relative "low point" in blood counts (WBC and platelets) following chemotherapy infusions. This measurement is crucial in timing and dosing chemotherapy because it correlates to the bone marrow's production of blood. The average nadir is ten days, but the precise nadir range is dependent on the drug given. At the low point, patients are more susceptible to infection and bleeding.

Central line: Delivery of chemotherapy can occur through a central line that is surgically placed into a vein in the chest.

Immunotherapy: Aptly referred to as biologic therapy because it enhances the body's own immune system to fight neoplastic disease. Substances made by the body or in laboratories are injected into the patient to stimulate stronger immune function.

Fundamental Terminology for Western Physicians

Diagnostics

Tongue: The tongue inspection is a unique and important diagnostic method in TCM and gives insight into the health of an individual. It is used to observe abnormal changes in the tongue body, such as color and shape as well as the quality and coloring of the tongue coating in order to analyze and diagnose disease.

Pulse: Pulse diagnosis is a major tool to help practitioners gain understanding into the pattern of disharmony at that moment in time. An acupuncturist will feel your pulse on the radial artery on both sides feeling the quality, depth and rhythm. The pulse can signify the thermal nature of a disease, assess the pathogenesis of a disease and reach a prognosis of disease.

Palpation: Utilizes the sense of touch to feel, press or palpate areas of the patient's body, including the pulse, abdomen and meridians in order to obtain information regarding the patient's physiological and pathological condition.

Inquiry: Practitioner engages in conversation to gain insight into the patient's condition. The patient's symptoms, the cause or predisposing factors of the disease, the history (onset, development and treatment) of the disease, the patient's living environment and personal relationships are all collected to assist in the naming of the disease or differentiation of the pattern.

Examination: A detailed inspection or study of the patient using diagnostic tools such as measuring blood pressure, height and weight or range of motion tests. TCM examination heavily involves interacting with the patient through various diagnostic methods that fall into broader categories of Inquiry, Listening, Smelling, Palpating, and Observation.

Observation: Utilizes the practitioner's senses to observe abnormal changes in the patient's spirit, complexion, tongue and appearance.

Treatments

Acupuncture: An acupuncture point can be one of over 360 specific points on the 14 major meridians of the body where a therapeutic modality (needles, acupressure, moxibustion, massage) can be applied. An acupuncture point has a specific therapeutic effect on the energy of the meridian or organ system. Acupuncture points often work in conjunction with one another to create balance in the body.

Moxibustion: The warming of acupuncture points using the herb mugwort (artemesia). Moxibustion is usually applied to a needle or indirectly over the skin until a warming sensation is felt.

Chinese dietary therapy: Food therapy is a mode of nutrition rooted in the five/six flavors and is used to treat and prevent disease using the energetic thermal nature and properties of food.

Manual therapy (*tui na, sotai*): Manual therapy is physical manipulation to treat musculoskeletal pain and disability. It most commonly includes kneading and manipulation of muscles, joint mobilization and joint manipulation.

Chinese herbal medicine: Herbal therapy includes plants, animals/animal parts and minerals used singly or most commonly in formulas to treat a condition.

Physical exercise (*qigong, tai chi*): A set of exercises including meditative and physical movements. Used to move *qi*, thereby maintaining and regaining physical, emotional and spiritual health. These forms of exercise are considered an important internal cultivation of *qi*.

TCM Concepts

***Qi*:** Translates to "vital breath" or life force. In TCM, *qi* is believed to regulate a person's physical, emotional, mental and spiritual balance and to be influenced by the opposing forces of *yin* and *yang*. *Qi* is an organizing force, which includes many different types of *qi*, for example, Spleen *qi* or source *qi*, each have different roles and functions.

Blood: Blood is used as a broad term to describe the physical blood in the body that moistens the muscles, tissues, skin and hair, as well as nourishing the cells and organs.

Yin: A relative term in relation to *yang*, is associated with the more substantial parts of our body and of nature. *Yin* is associated with the material, feminine, nourishment, dark, moist, coolness, substantial and being rooted or grounded.

Yang: A relative term in relation to *yin* is associated with the more energetic parts of our body and nature. *Yang* is associated with function, masculine, energy, brightness, warmth, the ethereal, and rising up.

Jing/Essence: The substance responsible for reproduction. It is derived from the energy inherited from one's parents in combination with the energy a person acquires in daily life from air, food and water. *Jing/essence* regulates the body's growth and development, provides for reproductive health, and works with *qi* to help protect the body from harmful external factors.

Meridians/Channels: TCM utilizes a system of meridians identified by the ancient Chinese, through which vital substances, such as *qi* and blood, flow in the body. These meridians or channels are named for their organ system and are where the acupuncture points are organized.

Deficiency and Excess: Deficiency and excess are two principles and relative terms, which are used to distinguish the strength of the antipathogenic *qi* and the pathogenic factor. This clarification on whether a syndrome is deficiency or excess forms the basis for the treatment.

Damp-Phlegm: Excessive fluids in the body with symptoms of abdominal bloating, loss of appetite, nausea, vomiting, lack of thirst, feeling of heaviness or being sluggish, and stiff, aching or sore joints. Damp-phelgm occurs when the digestive function is impaired and can be generated internally or acquired externally.

Toxic Heat: Toxic heat is extreme heat in the system that can move more deeply and into all systems of the body. Typical hallmarks of toxic heat that differentiate it from other forms of heat are pain and often times, pus (e.g. skin boil). Toxic heat can often be a side-effect of chemotherapy treatment.

Stagnation/Stasis: Stagnation is a blockage or build-up of *qi*, blood or phlegm that prevents it from flowing freely. It is a precursor of illness and disease and can lead to lumps or masses.

Case Study Oncology Intake

Traditional Chinese medicine integrated oncology intake

Case History: A 54-year-old woman identified a firm, immobile lump in her left breast during self-breast exam. No prior cancer history or known family history.

Diagnosis: Breast Cancer Stage II — Left

I. Diagnostics

Western:	*TCM:*
Imaging: Mammogram, ultrasound, MRI	**Diagnosis**: Liver and Kidney *Yin* Deficiency with *Qi* Stagnation
Biopsy: Left breast, lymph node	**Tongue:** Dusky with a dry, thin white coat, red tip
Surgical: Mastectomy with implant expander for reconstruction; lymph node dissection	**Pulse**: *Chi* positions weak-thin; *Guan* positions wiry; Heart floating
Histopathology: Estrogen/ progesterone positive (ER/PR+) HER-2 neu negative	**Observation:** Surgical scar from mastectomy is pink-red, no visible swelling, range of motion is within normal ranges (arm extension and lateral raises)
Tumor size: 2.6 cm	**Palpation:** Surgical zone slightly warm, with acute scar tissue formation that is palpable and soft
Tumor Markers: BRCA 1–2 — negative	**Hara Abdominal Diagnosis:** Cool Spleen and soft Kidney, Stomach and Liver tight

II. Integrative Treatments

Western:	TCM:
External Radiotherapy x 5 weeks, 5 days/week Tamoxifen x 2–3 years until estrogen levels drop with menopause onset, then continue hormone therapy with aromatase-inhibitor (AI) x 2 years Breast reconstruction: Follow-up scheduled with surgical oncologist six months after completion of radiation therapy to determine breast health and surgery date.	**Acupuncture and Moxibustion Therapy:** • Post-Operative: Tonify *Qi* and Blood, Nourish *Yin*, Clear Excess Heat (surgical scar), Calm Spirit • Radiation Support: Clear Excess Heat, Relieve Toxicity, Nourish *Yin*, Generate Fluids **Chinese Herbal Medicine:** • Immune Support: *Cordyceps, Ren Shen, Huang Qi* • Radiation Therapy: topical burn cream applied twice per day after radiation exposure and before bed • Harmonize body's response to hormone therapy (Tamoxifen) to lessen intensity of menopausal syndrome symptomatology; base formula *Liu Wei Di Huang Wan* modified with herbs to regulate Liver *qi* and settle the spirit **Exercise:** • During radiation, eliminate running to avoid movement of breast implant. • Moderate walking • 2–3x/week barre classes • Emphasize grounding "*yin-exercise*" and morning/evening meditation

III. Cancer-Related Conditions & Potential Side Effects

Western:

Post-operative: local inflammation, pain local to surgical site, limited range of motion of left-shoulder

Radiation: local erythema of skin, peeling, itching, swollen, dry, possible ulcerations and acute pain, sensation of heat in affected area

Hormonal Side Effects due to Tamoxifen: insomnia, night sweats, hot flashes, mood changes, vaginal dryness, tendency toward anxiety and depression

IV. Supportive Therapeutic Recommendations

Dietary Advice:

Patient's diet is clean, already gluten-free, minimal to no dairy intake, processed foods or sugar.

Recommended: 1–2 cups of bone broth daily; during radiation avoid raw, uncooked, cold foods that inhibit Spleen/Stomach ability to digest and build blood (*yin* substance) because radiation depletes *yin*. Decrease intake of spicy food (too hot in nature) and include *yin*-nourishing foods.

Professional Referrals:

Oncology Dietician — for more detailed assessment of nutritional guidelines

Physical Therapist — to assess mobility of left breast, underarm and shoulder to optimize healing and avoid cording or fibrosis

TCM Treatment Plan:

During radiation: weekly acupuncture therapy and moxibustion

Tamoxifen: modified herbal prescription for hormonal support according to constitution

There are no absolutes in the treatment of cancer. The disease is naturally elusive, keen on being mysterious and challenging rather than cooperative. Western medicine can meet the demands of the disease. Both are aggressive, stalwart and motivated, fast-moving and in a biomedical sense, equally prepared for one another. At this point in modern medicine with regards to epidemics like cancer, we must rely upon established methods to eradicate unhealthy cells. But what about the healthy organisms? The ones trying to survive amidst the turmoil of disease and treatment? Herein lies the proverbial bridge, the pathway that unites the West to the East. This link recalibrates the way in which the individual navigating the vast realm of cancer is seen, heard and treated. It also broadens the avenue of integrative care.

In the preceding chapters each individual pillar of Chinese medicine was presented in order to demonstrate its therapeutic range in cancer management, prevention and recovery. Without a doubt, there are countless methods within this scope. The compilation of diagnostic methods and technique applications are derived from classical teachings, mentors and extensive clinical practice, which we recognize is exactly that, a practice. As medicine and illness evolve, so do the doctors. In that same vein, we humbly contribute our material, while knowing and expecting that our knowledge continues to build as we always retain the label of student. This is reflected in a statement by Mao Tse-tung on the importance of practice, "Knowledge begins with experience — this is the materialism of the theory of knowledge. Knowledge begins with practice, and theoretical knowledge is acquired through practice and must then return to practice."[235]

This preparation does not come easily. There are limited resources for the Chinese medicine profession in the subject of oncology. The available academic translations from our colleagues in Asia are valuable contributions, but not all of the therapeutic applications can be adapted to Western medical systems. It is challenge enough integrating moxibustion therapy into clinical settings, much less herbal prescription. We hope the influence from our colleagues at hospitals abroad who have successfully integrated conventional oncology with Chinese medicine for decades inspires the West. Until then, TCM is resolute in its capacity to translate biomedical components into Chinese medical interventions. It continues to examine the physiological terrain, relative to the disease process, observing singular interactions as parts to a greater whole. To thoroughly

---

[235] Unschuld, 1985

illustrate the essence of integration, mutual relationships and collaborative interactions is the following quote, intended for doctors of New Medicine in 20th century China:

> "The parts and the whole together form a relationship, in which they oppose one another, but yet at the same time constitute homogenous entity. If there are no parts, there is also no whole, if there is no whole, there are also no parts. In therapy it is not permissible to concentrate solely on the partial factor of pathological changes, losing sight of the whole process, such as in the case of a headache to treat only the head, or in the case of foot pains to treat only the foot. Similarly, one cannot view only the whole and ignore the partial factor of pathological changes, by carrying out a general course of treatment of the entire body while neglecting, at the same time, the individual elements of the nidus. The correct approach is as follows: Proceed from a consideration of the whole; concentrate not only on the parts but put an even greater emphasis on the entire situation, combining both aspects dialectically. In this manner, a treatment of the parts can be implemented that will also influence the entire body; moreover, a treatment of the entire body can be carried out in such a manner that will, at the same time, affect the parts."[236]

The evolution of modern medical disciplines is a byproduct of thousands of years of practice. The phases of learning explored layers of the body that encompass the whole person such as anatomy and the cellular profile, channels and the energetic systems within them. These mutual relationships correspond to wellness and disease, identified through the Western and Eastern medical lens. These are interconnected systems, singular parts to a complete whole, intended to potentiate the effects of the other. Conventional oncology and traditional Chinese medicine

---

[236] Unschuld, 1985

intrinsically collaborate. Balanced integration is possible. This is the time for new medicine.

References

Abrams, D., Mcculloch, M., Cohen, M., Liaw, M., Silverman, D., & Wilson, C. (2018). A Survey of Licensed Acupuncturists in the San Francisco Bay Area: Prevalence of Treating Oncology Patients. *Integrative Cancer Therapies,17*(1), 92–98. doi:10.1177/1534735416684946

Seely, D. (2012). *A systematic review of integrative oncology programs.* Retrieved July 10, 2014, from current-oncology.com: http://www.currentoncology.com/index.php/oncology/article/view/1182/1078

Servan-Schreiber, D. (2009). *Anticancer: A New Way of Life.* New York, NY: Viking.

Unschuld, P. U. (1985). *Medicine in China: A History of Ideas.* Berkeley, California: University of California Press.

Index